The Message
of
GRACE

The Message of GRACE

A Bible Study by Wayne A. Barber

DISCIPLESHIP SERIES

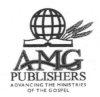

AMG
PUBLISHERS
ADVANCING THE MINISTRIES
OF THE GOSPEL

Following God
Message of Grace

© 2016 by Wayne Barber

ISBN: 978-0-89957-336-6
First Printing, 2016

Cover design by Daryl Phillips, Chattanooga, TN
Editing by Trevor Overcash, Joy Rankin and Rick Steele, Jr.

Typesetting and page layout by Jennifer Ross

Printed in the United States of America
20 19 18 17 16 15 –AZ– 6 5 4 3 2 1

CONTENTS

I first met Wayne Barber at a home Bible fellowship in the 1980's, and we hit it off immediately. His message of grace resonated with what God was doing in my life, and the friendship was formative for me. I was in ministry in another town, but every time I would visit Chattanooga, we would get together for lunch and talk Scripture. His faith and trust was contagious, and I am grateful God brought him into my life so early in my early ministry years. He often would say that he would love to have me on his church staff one day, and in 1989 that became a reality. I am so grateful for the many years God allowed me to co-labor with him and be impacted by his leadership and heart for God.

Under Wayne's leadership in those days, Woodland Park Baptist Church had grown from 150 members to 1500 in less than a decade. People from all over the region were attracted to his message of grace, his rich Bible teaching, and his humble, self-effacing humor. It was a formative time for Wayne as well. He began teaching weekly with Kay Arthur and Precept Ministries, and began co-hosting a television and radio program called "New Testament Light" with eminent Greek scholar, Spiros Zodhiates. Both friendships deepened his Bible teaching even more.

Wayne Barber, Rick Shepherd and I used to joke that the "Following God" Bible study series we authored together was born "somewhere over Greenland." The three of us were flying back to the U.S. from training pastors in Romania, and as we reflected on what we felt had been most effective, the character sketches seemed to have the greatest impact. Over the next year, we wrote several Bible studies and piloted them at our church with a view to translating them into Romanian for the next pastor's conference. Our primary goal was Bible study resources for Romania. It didn't occur to us that they might have a broader appeal, but when AMG Publishers got wind of what we did at our church, they approached us about publishing the studies and the rest is history.

This latest installment in the Following God® series was a lifetime in the making. It was truly Wayne Barber's life message. Although the bulk of writing was completed four years ago, this project was circumstantially delayed, and a week and a half before his unexpected passing, AMG Publishers announced its scheduled release was set for two months later. As Wayne would say, "God is good all the time, right on time, just in time....Why? Because that's His nature!" Although he is in heaven now, his ministry continues. My prayer is that this message of grace would transform your life and walk, as it has mine.

Eddie Rasnake

Co-author Following God® Bible studies series
Woodland Park Baptist Church, Chattanooga, Tennessee

TO
my wife, Diana
my daughter, Stephanie Christensen
and
my son, Stephen Barber
only heaven will tell how much I love each of you!

PREFACE

One day a farmer was showing his grandson his multi acre farm. The farmer took the boy all around, pointing out the big red barn, the beautiful horses and the golden fields of corn. As they were walking, the grandson noticed something unusual on the horizon. There was a big, strong looking man pumping a well. This was unusual in that this man pumped hard and fast, never once stopping to catch his breath or wipe his brow. The little boy's curiosity got the best of him, and he finally said, "Grandpa, where did you find a man who could pump a well like that?" The old farmer chuckled and said, "Son, that's an Artesian well! That man is not real, but wooden and he is not pumping that well, the well is pumping him!" Sure enough as they got closer, the grandson could see that the strong, muscular arms were nothing more than thick pieces of timber bolted together in the form of a man. The fresh water flowing was not a result of a man's hard effort, but of a cleverly built machine that moved the wooden man, causing the work to be done.

Do you ever feel like you are trying to be that wooden man? You sweat and strive to get the work done, yet the only fruit of your labor is exhaustion and pain. The Bible tells us to cease striving and know that He is God. Isn't that a beautiful thought? Cease striving. Think about that for a moment. Many of us have never contemplated that thought before when it comes to our Christian life. When I stop and contemplate it, only one word can come to my mind and that is *grace*! God's Grace! Like that Artesian well, God comes to live in me to do in and through me what I could never do on my own.

Grace is a marvelous subject that could never be exhausted in one study. Although grace has the distinction of being in the title of many of our churches and the subject of most of the hymns we sing, very few of us understand what it is all about and how to apply it to everyday life. All of God's goodness is found in grace. All that we have in and because of Christ is housed in that one little word. Many well-meaning believers have wandered away from "grace" and have strayed back under the performance mentality of the "law." They have fallen into a religious trap and as a result, they are burned out, bitter, discouraged, critical, and wondering if they were ever even saved in the first place. How and what they do at church has become their only way to measure their spirituality, and they have no intimacy with Christ in their daily walk. Many times these deceived believers are the very ones who stand at the doors of the church and greet others outwardly with a gracious smile and an outstretched arm, while inwardly they are overcome with frustration and defeat. Their lives are empty, and they are afraid to honestly share their lack of joy for fear of being judged as "unspiritual."

It is to these discouraged pilgrims that this study has been written. As one who once lived in this same frustration, my prayer is that God would encourage you as you study the Scriptures and teach you the wondrous meaning of His grace and how it can affect every aspect of your life.

LESSON 1

GRACE: EXPERIENCING THE POWER OF THE CHRIST LIFE

What do you think about when you think of the Apostle Paul? Paul gives a pretty compelling biography of himself in Philippians 3:5-6. He was *"circumcised the eighth day, of the nation of Israel, of the tribe of Benjamin, a Hebrew of Hebrews; as to the law, a Pharisee, as to zeal, a persecutor of the church, as to the righteousness which is in the law, found blameless."* That's a pretty amazing background, yet when Paul assesses his own life, he counts all of this as loss for the sake of Jesus Christ.

"For to me, to live is Christ, and to die is gain." Philippians 1:21

This week we are going to take a fascinating look at the life of Paul and the letter he wrote to the church at Philippi. Paul understood something that would change our lives if we could just get a hold of it. What enabled Paul to *"count all things as loss"*? What was it that made Paul tick? Paul says in Philippians 1:21, *"for to me to live is Christ, and to die is gain."* Christ was the essence of Paul's very life, and as you study you will see what a difference this truth can make.

Our English word *"grace"* in the Bible is translated from the word *charis* in the Greek language. According to the *Complete Word Study New Testament* by Spiros Zodhiates, it is "particularly that which causes joy, pleasure, gratification, favor, and acceptance, for a kindness granted or desired, a benefit, thanks, and gratitude. It is favor done without expectation of return; the absolutely free expression of the loving kindness of God to men finding its only motive in the bounty and benevolence of the Giver; unearned and unmerited favor. *Charis* stands in direct antithesis to the Greek word *erga*, meaning 'works,' and the two being mutually exclusive. God's grace affects man's sinfulness and not only forgives the repentant sinner, but also brings joy and thankfulness to him. It is the transforming power of God that changes the individual to a new creature without destroying his individuality (2 Cor. 5:17; Eph. 2:8-9)."

> *God's grace affects man's sinfulness and not only forgives the repentant sinner, but also brings joy and thankfulness to him.*

In this lesson we are going to study a man who obviously understood and lived in the riches of God's grace. This man is the apostle Paul. A man who was raised under "law," even to the point of being taught by the greatest teacher of the Law during his time, named Gamaliel. It is interesting to note that when the apostles were brought before the council, charged with preaching the resurrection of Jesus, Gamaliel, as a righteous Pharisee, counseled moderation and calmness. By a reference to well known events, he advised the Sanhedrin to "refrain from these men." If their work or counsel was of man, it would come to nothing, but if it was of God they could not destroy it, and therefore ought to be on their guard lest they should be "found fighting against God" (see Acts 5:34-40). Paul was once one of Gamaliel's disciples. Open your Bible now to the book of Philippians and let's begin our journey in understanding the practical message of "grace" as we look at this man who was totally changed by it and learned to live in it daily.

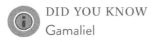 DID YOU KNOW
Gamaliel

Gamaliel was the son of Rabbi Simeon, and grandson of the famous Rabbi Hillel. He was a Pharisee, and therefore opponent of the party of the Sadducees. He was noted for his learning, and president of the Sanhedrin during the reigns of Tiberius, Caligula, and Claudius. It is said that he died about 18 years before the destruction of Jerusalem.

Day 1

Prison Time

There are many questions to ask in studying a book of Scripture. Although we are not going to study the entire book of Philippians in detail, we need to ask some of these questions so that we can get a look into the circumstances in Paul's life as he writes to the church at Philippi. In chapter 1, there are quite a few verses that give us an indication of where Paul is when he writes.

Read through the first chapter of Philippians and answer the following questions.

Where is Paul when he writes this letter?

_____

_____

According to the following verses, what single word in each verse gives an indication of where Paul is when he writes this letter?

Philippians 1:7 _____

Philippians 1:13 _____

Philippians 1:14 _____

Philippians 1:17 _____

Now read Acts 21:17 through Acts 28:31. I know this is a lot of reading, but it will give you a good background in understanding the circumstances that put Paul in prison. Note what you learn about Paul's situation. Was his prison a result of sin on his part?

_____

_____

DAILY REFLECTION

Paul was writing this letter under house arrest. He was in prison for more than five years for something he didn't even do. What a blessing to read through this chapter and see how Paul responded to this trial in his life. In Day 2 we will begin to look at why Paul was able to respond in this way. Do you find yourself in a prison right now? Are you going through a difficult time as a result of your obedience to God? God never promised it would be easy, but He did promise He would be with us. He wants to empower you with His message of grace. Write out a prayer to Him now. Even if it is out of desperation, Psalms says that God will not despise a broken and a contrite heart (Psalm 51:17).

Day Two

Christ Is My Life

What does it mean for Christ to be your life? Paul certainly understood this and applied it to his life. Before we delve into this truth, let's first review some practical helps in Bible study. It is important when studying God's Word that we make certain to observe the text. As we saw yesterday in understanding Paul's circumstance in writing Philippians, the context should always be the foundation. There are three basic factors that must be considered when studying God's Word.

Observation – coming to an understanding of what the text says

Interpretation- coming to an understanding of what the text means

Application – coming to a practical understanding of how to adjust your life to the truths gleaned from observation and interpretation

It is important when studying God's Word that we make certain to observe the text.

In observing a passage of Scripture, it is always helpful to first read through it and then note the repeated words or phrases. This information helps you develop a theme of the chapter and/or book that is being studied. After observing the text of Philippians, many people conclude that "rejoice" or "joy" is the theme of the book. Now let's see if this is so.

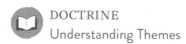 EXTRA MILE:
Some Keywords in the book of Philippians are:

Jesus, Christ, and Lord
Joy, Rejoice,
Attitude, Mind
If you see any other repeated words or phrases that bear importance on the meaning of the text, write them here.

_____

_____

Read through the book of Philippians. As you read, note how many times each of the following words or phrases are used. You may want to mark them in a specific color.

1) Jesus, Christ, and Lord in any and all combinations _____

2) Joy, Rejoice _____

3) Attitude, Mind _____

As you can see, the name of Christ is mentioned so many times that we can easily conclude that He is the theme of this book! The words "joy" and "rejoice" are used enough times to be a sub theme, as are attitude and mind.

Once you find the theme of the book, you begin to notice how the chapters are put together and how they flow together to bring out the theme. Chapter titles help immensely not only in remembering the chapter content, but also seeing how the theme is brought out in the book.

DOCTRINE
Understanding Themes

Developing titles and themes to a text of Scripture helps you get a handle on what the author is saying. You could say it's like a carrying a suitcase. The handle makes it easier for you to carry what is contained within the suitcase. So it is with God's Word.

Read through the book of Philippians again giving a brief title for each chapter. Don't feel like you have to spend a lot of time on this; just write in a few words that you feel would best sum up the content of the chapter.

Chapter 1

_____

_____

Chapter 2

_____

_____

Chapter 3

_____

_____

Chapter 4

_____

_____

Now that you have a good overview of the four chapters in Philippians, you have probably seen the theme of Paul's life and of this letter to the church of Philippi. It is Philippians 1:21. Write out this verse below.

_____

_____

_____

> _"In Philippians 1:21, the word "life" is translated from the Greek zoé. It is used to describe the very essence of life."_

For centuries man has debated over the two complex issues of life and death, and here Paul sums them both up in one verse! The word "life" in this verse is translated from the Greek _zoe_. It is the word describing the essence of _life_. Look up the following verses and note what you learn from each one about the word _life_.

1) John 10:10

_____

_____

2) John 3:16

_____

_____

3) Romans 5:9 (Notice whose life it is that not only saved us, but also saves us daily).

_____

_____

4) Colossians 3:4

_____

_____

Christ is our life! That is the key to understanding the message of Grace. Now that you know that Paul is in prison when he writes this letter, how do you think this mentality changed his whole perspective towards his circumstances?

_____

_____

_____

Look at Philippians 1:12-13. The Praetorian Guard has to do not only with the soldiers that were Caesar's elite, but also their headquarters there in Rome. Isn't it interesting that in order for God to get the gospel to Caesar's very household he had to make certain that Paul was in chains? So often we kick against the very things that God is using to reach those that we could have never touched otherwise. God squeezed out of Paul the message that they needed to hear. Did it work? Look at chapter 4:22. What do you observe?

_____

_____

_____

"So often we kick against the very things that God is using to reach those that we could have never touched otherwise."

DAILY REFLECTION

What does this say to you and me about allowing Christ to be our life in the midst of very uncomfortable and unkind circumstances?

_____

_____

_____

_____

"Christ is my life therefore prisons don't defeat me!"

How are you dealing with the prisons in your life? It is no mistake that God has you doing this study during this time in your life. How does He want to speak to you in His Word? Take some time and meditate on what you learned today. If you sense God encouraging you in any way, write it down. It will be a great source of strength to you in the future when you look back at how God brought you through a difficult time. Do you feel distant from God? Is there an attitude or sin that has you hiding from His presence? A beloved friend and mentor of mine once told me that no matter how far away you may feel from

God, the distance back to Him is only as far as it is for you to get on your knees. Be quiet in your heart before God and let Him minister His truth to you.

DAY THREE

CHRIST IS MY ATTITUDE

In chapter one we found that "Christ is our life" (Phil. 1:21). Understanding this truth causes us to have a different perspective when it comes to "prisons" He allows in our lives (Philippians 1:12-14). Are you starting to see how practical the message of grace can be in your daily life? When Christ is living His life in and through us, we are suddenly able in His grace to "deal" with life's circumstances. As you will see throughout the rest of this week, when this truth is applied it begins to filter out into every area of our lives. Now in chapter 2 of Philippians, Paul's focus moves from prisons to people.

> *"When Christ is living His life in and through us, we are suddenly able in His grace to "deal" with life's circumstances."*

Read through chapter 2 paying close attention to verses 1–4.

Write out verse one.

Let's go through verse 1 and look at the meaning of it word by word.

If - this word can be translated from the Greek as "since." This means that it is a certainty. It's no longer "if there is," but "since there is."

encouragement - *parakaleō*. This means to "come alongside" and "to encourage."

consolation - *paramuthion*. This differs somewhat from encouragement. It means to verbalize comfort to someone. The first is the desire to come alongside for the sake of encouragement, whereas the second involves the words that one would use to do just that.

fellowship of the Spirit – This seems to have the meaning of "spiritual fellowship." It refers to that which is caused by the Spirit of God living in us. Christ's Spirit (the

Holy Spirit) lives within us. He produces a "fellowship" (the word means a participation, a sharing in) that we can all partake of together.

affection – This literally refers to the "bowels" of something. It is used figuratively as the inward caring one has for others. This is the deep love that God produces in a believer for those in the Body of Christ.

compassion – *oiktimos*. This is similar to our word "mercy" but has some differences. It refers to the deep compassion and pity one has for those who are suffering.

Think about these characteristics in relation to your church and spiritual friendships. Reflect for a moment on the importance of each quality to be present in these relationships. Look back at verse 1 again. Where does it say that all of these characteristics are found? Where do we find the ability and the desire to build these characteristics in our lives?

*"Christ is the well that we draw from
in order for us to be of service to others."*

In Christ! He is the well that we draw from in order for us to be of service to others. Let me go one step further. Can we work this lifestyle up in our own ability? Can a church truly be characterized by these qualities simply as a result of human ingenuity? NO! This is found only in Christ! In fact, all that we need in our relationships with others we already have in Christ, who is our life.

With that in mind, let's read on and watch what Paul does. Read verse 2. It is to this purpose of seeing others as Christ sees them and to minister to them in His ability that we all must come to. We must all have this same mind, or attitude, towards one another.

Read the first part of verse 3. Are there other motivations that cause believers to do what they do in regard to others in the Body of Christ?

*"Do nothing out of selfishness or empty conceit,
but with humility of mind let each of you regard one another
as more important than himself"*

Philippians 2:3

Note the phrase, *"do nothing from selfishness or empty conceit."* The word *nothing* means absolutely NOTHING! The word *selfishness* means, "that which comes out of a person who has only selfish intentions." Think for a minute. Can people actually serve others out of a selfish motivation? Well, the next phrase, *empty conceit*, is a word that means "a desire for personal praise." What does this tell you?

_____

_____

_____

Paul has already told us of the motivation of some people who "preach Christ" Go back to Philippians 1:15. The Greek word translated "strife" in Philippians 1:15 is a synonym for the word translated "selfishness" here in Philippians 2:3 (NASB).

Having studied this, what should our motivation in serving others be, and what is its source when it comes to all our relationships?

_____

_____

_____

The motivation and its source is Christ, who is our life!

> *"What we do, we do in His power and our motivation comes from Him and not our own selfish intentions."*

Now, in Lesson 2, He becomes our attitude towards others. What we do, we do in His power, and our motivation comes from Him and not our own selfish intentions. He changes the way we see others just as He changes the way we look at the circumstances in life.

How has Christ affected the way you look at others?

_____

_____

_____

Verse 5 is the focus and pivotal verse in this chapter.

Philippians 2:5 *"Have this attitude in yourselves which was also in Christ Jesus. . . ."*

> *Christ is my attitude therefore people don't bother me.*

Read verses 6-11. Write down your understanding of how this relates to our attitude towards others. Note the attitude of Christ who is and always will be God! What is our attitude to be towards others?

_____

_____

_____

_____

DAILY REFLECTION

Well friend, are you seeing how directly your attitude is affected when Christ is your life? When He is your life, He also becomes your attitude. Are you frustrated with people today? I used to say that the Christian life would be easy if it weren't for people! What we need to remember when it comes to relationships is that we cannot love the way God intends us to love! Remember what you read in Philippians 2:1. This type of love is only found in Christ! He must be your life before He can be your attitude. Let Him be your life by surrendering to Him afresh right now. You will be surprised at how your attitude will change because the love that He will work in you is a love not of yourself, but of God. Let God fill you with His love today. Take some time to reflect on your relationships. Meditate on chapter two. Ask God to do in and through you what you could never do on your own.

_____

_____

_____

_____

_____

_____

_____

_____

_____

_____

_____

_____

_____

DAY FOUR

GOD USES RELIGION AND LEGALISM TO BRING US TO HIM

When you look carefully at the epistles in the New Testament that were written by the apostle Paul you can tell he looked at all the people as the same, sinners saved by grace. Flesh is the same for everyone and is the same everywhere. We have already learned that our relationships are not able to flourish if we are walking according our own flesh and unwilling to put that flesh to death. Often we can see how God allows us to have our taste of religion when we want it. For many of us it's easier to have the rituals without the relationship.

God is only impressed when He looks at us and sees Himself

Philippians chapter 3 we learn about Paul's former life in "religion." Let's examine verse 1. The word for "rejoice" is in the present tense ("keep on rejoicing"). Paul had felt the need to write this letter to the church at Philippi to remind them to rejoice even in the face of struggle and hardship.

In verse 2 Paul gives a stern warning about the "religious." Essentially Paul is cautioning against following those whose motivations are not from God but from the flesh. The dogs mentioned here refer to the religious leaders, those who led those that followed to be under the bondage of the Law. Remember here that the Philippian believers were members of a Gentile church and thus were not Jews. Paul is "flipping the script" and uses the language that was typically used to describe Gentiles to describe his "own kind."

What are some of the ways that we tend to follow after those that establish rules?

_____

_____

DOCTRINE
In the New Testament, many references are made to "dogs." Many passages include this word to describe those from Gentile ethnic groups. However, in this Philippians 3 passage, the dogs here are referring to the group Paul used to be part, specifically the religious elite. The focus of these religious groups is to put people back up under the Law instead of grace.

During the time that Paul (Saul) was persecuting the church, he believed that those who followed Jesus Christ were rejecting the Law and should be destroyed. But as a follower of Jesus himself Paul learned about the "true circumcision" (Phil. 3:3). Now, Paul has learned that these "efforts" were futile and our focused has turned from ourselves to bringing God glory.

Read verse 3. How does Paul describe his own flesh when it comes to worshiping God?

_____

_____

Paul states clearly here that he has no confidence in his own flesh to do anything for God. Now examine how Paul explains his lack of confidence in his own flesh. Verses 4-6 give us a detailed description of how Paul was "qualified" in man's view to have "confidence in his flesh before God. List the difference ways that Paul qualified himself (verses 5, 6):

_____

_____

_____

The legalists of Paul's day put a lot of importance on their birth, their heritage, their pedigree and their accomplishments. As far as the Jews were concerned, Paul met the requirements. He was "circumcised on the eighth day," which made his heritage. He was from the tribe of Benjamin. His heritage could be traced back and he knew his family line. He was a Pharisee and a very devout and committed one. His commitment led him to be part of the group that persecuted followers of Jesus Christ, putting many to death including Stephen (Acts 7:58-8:1).

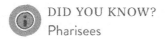 DID YOU KNOW?
Pharisees

A Pharisee was a member of a religious sect of Judaism. Representatives of this group were spokesmen for the Law. There were many examples of conflicts and conversations between Jesus and members of this group during the time He was on this earth. John chapter 3 recounts a conversation Jesus had with Nicodemus, a noted Pharisee, where Jesus lovingly confronted his false beliefs.

Paul summarized his evaluation of the "qualifications" he listed to make him religious (verse 7) by referring to those accomplishments as "loss" for the sake of Christ. Paul was rejecting those things that in the eyes of those around him made him successful. He further explains in verse 8 that "all things" that he could do, even for Christ's sake are to be counted as loss in order to know Christ more fully, which is ultimately gain. In verse 9 Paul reminds the Philippians again that his own righteousness was found in the Law before, but now is found in God through faith in Christ.

Paul lived every day to see God enable Paul
to bear up under his circumstances

In verse 10 Paul explains that the faith to become righteous in God's eyes through the work of Jesus has a practical, daily result. Paul desired to "know Him" and to live each day through the power God provides. The English word for "know" in Philippians 3:10 comes from the Greek word *ginosko*, meaning, "to know him experientially." This means that God produces in us a love for others even when they are unlovable. He goes on to emphasize this in two ways. Read verse 10 and list the ways that Paul could experience "knowing Him":

_____

_____

_____

_____

Paul was sharing a simple truth: he wanted to be called the "living" among the dead. Those that followed religious rituals were not truly alive, but those who lived under grace can experience all that it means to be alive in Christ.

DAILY REFLECTION

God places many of us in places where there is no light so that we can be light among those who have not experienced God's light. Once you have experienced this for yourself, you start to recognize what God is doing in your life and how much those around us desperately need us. Won't you take a moment and pray asking God to show you what you have experienced in your walk with Him that you can share with others? Write down any thoughts that come to your mind that you can ask God to strengthen in your heart.

_____

_____

_____

_____

_____

_____

_____

_____

DAY FIVE

THE SOURCE OF OUR STRENGTH

As we have studied together, we can see the key verse in chapter 1 is verse 21. In chapter 2, the key verse can be seen as verse 5 (having the mind of Christ). In chapter 3, we see that Paul's goal was to remain in a relationship with God that so glorified Him. In chapter 4, Paul sums up all that he has been teaching the Philippian church.

Read Philippians 4:13. Summarize what Paul shares as the source for any power a believer possesses:

_____

_____

Paul describes the blessing he had received from the gift the church in Philippi sent to him in his time of need (Phil. 4:10,11). It was not a need that Paul expressed to them directly, but they were able to provide it to him nonetheless. As Paul recounts that blessing, he reminded those believers that he had found true contentment. The word for contentment used in verse 11 has the meaning of being "self-contained." He was not in need because all he needed was found in Christ.

Jesus be Jesus in me. No longer me, but Thee.

The key element to all that Paul was seeking to encourage the Philippian believers, and even to us today, is to allow Jesus to be Jesus in us. The best example I can give to illustrate this truth is the one of a coat. When I go to the store and I see a coat hanging on the hanger, I can command it to come to me, but it cannot move or do anything by itself. I can ask the sleeve to wave at me, but it does not have the ability. It does not have life of its own. That coat hangs on the coat rack at the store, destined to rot until someone comes and picks it up and puts it on and redeems it. Once I am wearing the coat, it moves at my will. It has my life inside it.

What this illustrates is that law can never produce what it demands (Romans 7). The only way that the coat comes to life is for Jesus to get inside the coat, or inside of us. He redeemed us at a high price. He offers a life that is better than anything the Law provides. John 10:10 says, "I have come that you might have life, and have it more abundantly."

> *Religion demands what we cannot produce. When Jesus gets inside*
> *you, you have all you need, and then you are truly alive in Him.*

DAILY REFLECTION

Is your hope in what you can try to produce yourself or in the One who lives inside you? Ask Him to show you areas in your life where you are not fully surrendered to Christ. Pray and ask God to help you each day to live in His strength and in His power.

LESSON 2

LIVING UNDER GRACE

We have seen very clearly the life of a man who understood what it meant to live under grace. In Lesson One, we saw that Paul was in prison in Rome, yet all he could talk about was his Christ. Christ was his life; Christ was his attitude; Christ was his goal, and Christ was his strength. Would you like to understand more about how to live this way? Paul wrote an epistle to the Romans several years before he was imprisoned and arrived in Rome. Martin Luther said that if the whole Bible were a ring, then the epistle of Romans would be the setting of that ring. This wonderful letter of Paul to the Romans is called the constitution of our faith. It explains more clearly the difference between Christianity and religion than any other place in Scripture.

> *"If the whole Bible was a ring, then the epistle of Romans would be the setting of that ring"*
>
> Martin Luther

You say, "I thought Christianity was a religion." Where did you get that? Religion is what man can do for God. And, the sad truth of that statement is that God has already condemned man's effort. During a flight a woman said to me, after she found out that I was a minister, "Religion never worked for me! I could never be good enough!" I said, "Praise the Lord, it never worked for me either." You see, the difference in Christianity and religion is in what God can do through a person. Christ comes to live in a believer and becomes that person's enabling power. Christ does through that person what he or she could never do alone.

> *Christ does through the believer what he could never do on his own!*

This week, we are going to look into this wonderful truth. Now remember as you study, that Paul is writing to believers in Rome. He wants them to understand the difference in the enabling power of God's grace in them and the performance mentality (which all religion demands) that most of them had towards their Christianity. Let's enter this glorious truth found in Romans 6.

Day 1

You Are Under Grace

The day this truth was revealed to me was a glorious day! I do not believe it is just taught; it has to be caught! Pray as you do your lesson homework today and ask God to reveal to you how He has set you free! Free indeed!

"So if the Son makes you free, you will be free indeed."

John 8:36

Look at Romans 6:14, *"For sin shall not be master over you, for you are not under law, but under grace."* Now look back at Romans 5:2, *"through whom also we have obtained our introduction by faith into this grace in which we stand; and we exult in hope of the glory of God."*

Paul says we stand _____ grace. We were introduced to this grace through_____

_____

Now, Romans 6:14 says, *"For sin shall not be master over you, for you are not under law, but _____ grace."*

The word *"under"* in this verse is translated from the Greek word *hupo. Hupo* states the condition or state in which we find every believer in Christ. We are no longer under the

_____.

We are under_____.

WORD STUDY
More on the Word "Under."

The Complete Word Study Dictionary New Testament gives a little more detail for the word hupo (translated "under" in Romans 6:14: Hupo (Strongs #5259) implies "being or remaining under a place or condition, . . . the Law (Rom 6:14-15; 1Co 9:20; Gal 4:3–5, Gal 4:21; Gal 5:18); the curse (Gal 3:10); the yoke (1Ti 6:1); grace (Rom 6:14–15). Figuratively of being under the power of something, e.g., sin, the law, the mighty hand of God, under His feet (Rom 7:14; Rom 16:20; 1Co 15:25, 1Co 15:27; Gal 3:22–23; Eph 1:22; 1Pe 5:6)."

In the context of Romans 6:14, to be under something is to be under the control-ling power of something. So, to be under the law means to be under the controlling, condemning power of the Law. Before we came to know Christ, we all were under law. We were left to ourselves to accomplish what God orders in His divine law, the Ten Commandments. The Law stood over us and condemned us in our every effort to achieve what it demanded. The first five commandments of the Ten Commandments deal with loving God, the second five deal with loving others. All men are failures in their attempts to live according to God's divine law. We cannot love God, and we cannot love others. None of us can measure up to what God commands. But, God has a cure!

Read Romans 8:2–4. The law (principle, or authority) of the Spirit (the One who gives us Life in Christ Jesus), "has set us free" from the law of sin and death.

What is the weakness of the Law found in verse 3?

_____

_____

The Law cannot produce what it demands because those to whom it is demanded suffer from the weakness of the flesh in their inability to produce it!

Look further in verse 3. How did God send His Son?

_____

_____

He _____ sin in the _____

Look at verse 4. Why would God send Jesus in the likeness of sinful flesh?

_____

_____

_____

Jesus met the requirements of the Law! Do you see what this means to us as believers? We can never meet God's standard of living. We cannot fulfill the requirements of the Law. But, because of Christ, the requirements of the Law have been met, and therefore the standard of God is satisfied because His Son now lives within us.

Because of Christ, how do we now walk? (verse 4)

_____

_____

_____

Now that the law has been met and fulfilled by the Perfect Man, we have a way through Christ to return to the relationship with God that was lost when Adam sinned. The way we enter is through Christ, who fulfilled the Law and paid our sin debt, as we trust Him and Him only to save us from our sin and to produce in and through us what He demands.

WORD STUDY
Dikaióō or Justification (Romans 5:1).

According to *The Complete Word Study Dictionary New Testament*, verbs which end in óō generally indicate bringing out that which a person is or that which is desired, but not usually referring to the mode in which the action takes place. In the case of dikaióō, it means to bring out the fact that a person is righteous.

Romans 5:1 says that *"Therefore having been justified by_____, we have _____ with God through our Lord Jesus Christ."* The word justified comes from the Greek word *dikaiōō*, which means to be acquitted. You could think of justification as "just as if you've never sinned." The blood of Christ has freed me from the penalty of sin and has caused all the enmity with God to be washed away forever. Now that we are saved, we are free from the penalty of sin. All this transformation happened the moment we placed our faith in Christ. But, oh the cost of having our sins washed away! It cost Jesus His life's blood shed for us on the cross.

But it didn't end at the cross, as there is another glorious truth to see here. He not only came to save us from the **penalty** of sin, but he also came to save us from the **power** of sin! You see, even though we are saved, God's divine law must be fulfilled. In our own power we still cannot fulfill His divine law. That's why Christ came to live in us through His Holy Spirit.

Hallelujah! Jesus lives in us to fulfill this law as we learn to surrender to Him. Remember that the divine law is made up of two sections:

Loving God with all our hearts

Loving our neighbor as ourselves

The fruit (which only He can produce) of His Spirit is love. When the Spirit bears His fruit of love in us, the last part of verse 23 says, *"against such there is no _____."*

> *"But the fruit of the Spirit is love, joy, peace, longsuffering, kindness, goodness, faithfulness, gentleness, self-control."*
>
> Galatians 5:22–23a

DAILY REFLECTION

What are your thoughts up to this point? Do you have a better understanding of what Christ did for us on the cross? Do you sense a "performance mentality" present within your heart? Oh Friend, let Christ minister His truth to you that you no longer have to perform for God. You can never meet His standard of expectation. Realize that the only person who could ever meet God's standard is His precious Son, Jesus Christ. God can set you free to allow Jesus to be who He is in and through you. Jesus is the only one that satisfies the requirement of the Law and because of what He did at the cross, He, by His Holy Spirit, now lives within us! Write your prayer of Thanksgiving for what Christ has done by dying for you.

_____

_____

_____

_____

_____

_____

DAY 2

SIN SHALL NOT BE MASTER OVER YOU

It is one thing to talk about being free from the power of sin, but it is another thing to live in that truth. From time to time some sort of sin dominates all of us. How can sin have power over us if we are free in Christ from its power? Think on this as you work through your study time today.

Look again at Romans 6:14. *"For sin shall not be master over you, for you are not under law but under grace."* What does it mean for sin to be master over you? Is that possible?

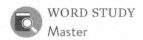

WORD STUDY
Master

The Greek word kúrios is found in the earliest manuscripts of the Book of Romans in several places when referring to things "as exercising mastery over us (Rom_6:9, Rom_6:14; Rom_7:1)." Kúrios is also used in the Septuagint (ancient Greek translation of the Old Testament in Judges 9:2 and Isaiah 19:4 and in both occurrences refers to rulers exercising dominion over subjects. (*The Complete Word Study Dictionary New Testament*) Our flesh always responds to the law's demand for performance either through rebellion or religion.

Paul speaks here of sin of any kind, and the Greek word translated *"master"* is *"kurieos,"* which means "to lord over, or to have authority over." "But wait a minute" you say, "sin from time to time does master me." Well, recognizing this is a good start! Thank you for being honest. Since we know this is the case, what is Paul trying to get across here? When you allow sin to master over you, you are essentially placing yourself back under the law. Law demands "performance." Our flesh responds to that demand for performance in one of two ways:

The first way is rebellion. Read Romans 1:18–32 and notice the rebellious side of the flesh. Although Paul is speaking of the pagan, Gentile world, flesh is flesh no matter which side of the cross you view it. It still wants to rebel.

The second way is religion. Read Romans 2:1—3:20 and notice here the proud, religious side of flesh as it responds to law.

> *Our flesh always responds to the law's demand for performance*
> *either through rebellion or religion.*

Who is Paul speaking to in chapter 2? Look at verse 1 and then verse 17. Whom does he address?

Religion is simply man's way of justifying his own external acts. Religion is a *"form of godliness,"* but it originates from man, not God. It is man's way of using God to parade his own abilities. God is not impressed. In fact, He has condemned every effort of man. Think of how we have all fallen into the trap of religion. What laws have we come up with that we think will justify ourselves before God? Consider this and make your list below.

Now that we have seen what it means to be "under law," we need to discover what it means to be "under grace." Let's go back to Romans 6 and see how Paul is able to say that we can be free from the dominion of sin in our lives.

In verses 1–5, Paul describes a brand new person in Christ. In verse 1, Paul addresses the group called the Antinomians. There were two groups of extremes in Rome. One were legalists who heard the grace message and could not stomach it; the other were the Antinomians." The prefix *anti* means against, while the root *nomos* means law. Unlike the legalists, the antinomians were the ones who mistakenly understood grace to mean free license to do whatever they wanted. They thought that since they were now under grace that their freedom included the right to do as they pleased. You see, true freedom does not give you the power to do as you please, but the power to do as you should! These Antinomians thought the more they sinned, the more grace they would receive. Do you know anyone like that today?

DID YOU KNOW?
More interesting Historical facts on Antinomians & legalists can be found at: outsidethecamp.org

Paul responds in verse 2 by saying, *"May it never be!"* Then he begins to build his case. *"How shall we who died to sin still live in it?"* Paul builds his case like a lawyer. He wants them to know that there has been a death. *"Or do you not know that all of us who have been baptized into Christ Jesus have been baptized into His death?"* (verse 3). Now, the word *baptize* is a word with two meanings. First is **immersion**, and second is **identification**. Both meanings are present in this verse. We have been **immersed** into Christ, but He has also come to live within us, and we are now **identified** with Him and all that He won for us on the cross. We are different than we were before we came to know Him.

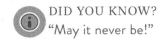
"May it never be!" is a phrase used at least 10 times in the book of Romans. It is a key phrase that expresses an absurdity to whatever is being talked about.

Paul continues to explain. Write verse 4 below.

_____

_____

_____

Christianity involves a death—death of what we used to be. And not only does it involve a death, but a resurrection. We are identified with His death when we are saved and also with His resurrection. He made us alive (Ephesians 2:1–3)! We have been raised to walk in the newness of His life. The word "new" means absolutely brand new—never before seen, qualitatively brand new. Everything to a believer is new. We must have our minds renewed with God's Word and learn to live in a totally different way. God wants us to walk in the newness of life.

> *Christianity not only involves a death of what we used to be, but a resurrection of His life in us!*

Paul continues with the thought in verse 5. *"For if we have become united with Him in the likeness of His death; certainly we shall be also in the likeness of His resurrection."* The word "united" is one of the most exciting words in this passage. It comes from the word *sumphutos*, originating from two Greek words: *sun*, which is the word for "with," and "*meta*" which means "by association." When one is part of a congregation on Sunday, he is "with" others (*meta*). Some can be added to the group, or some can leave, but the ones there are with each other for the time that they are in the service." But, this other word for "with," *sun*, is the one used here. This is the word that means to be with someone or some thing in an intimate, inseparable way. The verb form of *sumphutos* is the word *photos*, which conveys the idea of two things springing up together as one. Are you starting to see the special meaning that this little word puts into Romans 6:5? We were with him on the cross, and we are one with Him in His resurrection when we receive Him by faith. We are now united forever with His life. Inseparable.

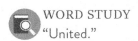

WORD STUDY

"United."

In Romans 6:5, the word "united" comes from the Greek *súmphutos*, which literally means to "grow together." In this verse, it conveys the idea of two plants "planted together, united with, innate." It also describes the oneness Christians "have with Christ in the likeness of His death, to be explained in accordance" with Romans 6:4 and 6:8. *Súmphutos* "denotes not merely homogeneousness, but a similarity of experience." (*The Complete Word Study Dictionary New Testament; súmphutos*, Strong's Greek # 4854.

DAILY REFLECTION

What a marvelous truth as we no longer have to allow sin to be the master over us. I like to think of sin like an evil slave driver cracking his whip! Thanks be to God who has delivered us through His Son Jesus Christ. Take a moment and think about your life. Do you find yourself under that slave driver's whip even though you know that you have been freed from sin's dominion through the blood of Christ? How can you know if you are allowing sin to have dominion over you? Well, for one thing, are you placing yourself back up under the dominion of laws trying to justify yourself before God? Do you sense rebellion in your life to the very truths that would set you free? We all have times where we allow our flesh to be the master over us. But, God has set us free from sin's dominion. Get quiet in your heart before the Lord and confess your weaknesses to Him. Let Him take control of the throne of your heart and free you now.

_____

_____

_____

_____

_____

_____

_____

_____

_____

_____

DAY 3

WHAT IS OUR PROBLEM?

We are brand new creatures when we receive Christ. Becoming a believer is much more than just joining a church! When we become believers in Christ, we become brand new creatures! Brand new! But, we now have a problem we never had. Romans 6:6 says, *"knowing this, that our old self was crucified with Him, that our body of sin might be done away with, that we should no longer be slaves to sin."* The Greek word translated *"knowing this"* suggests that this is a knowing that comes from experience. It doesn't take long for a believer to realize that, even though he is saved, there is a struggle that was not there before.

The term *"old self"* represents the "old person," basically who we were before we became Christians. What were we when we were in Adam (Romans 12:5)? We were *"devoid"* of the life of God when we were lost; there was no One living in us, drawing us towards the Father, no One living in us to convict us of sin and unrighteousness. But, when the Spirit of Christ, the Holy Spirit, comes to live in us, then we now have what we didn't have before, God's life in us. This is such an awesome truth! Jesus says in John 10:10, *"I have come that you might have life, and have it more abundantly."* The Christian life is much more than escaping hell. It starts with the realization that as lost people we don't have God's life in us. It is realizing that Jesus has come to give us life, to make us whole; the old self is dead.

> *"I have come that you might have life & have it more abundantly!"*
>
> John 10: 10

But, Paul continues in Romans 6:6, *"knowing this, that our old self was crucified with Him, that our body of sin might be done away with. . . ."*

Now, notice what Paul calls the body. The body of _____

_____

When you get up in the morning, you might remind yourself, "Good Morning, Body of Sin!"

Paul says that this body of sin might be *"done away with."* The word used here is *katargeo* (*kata* meaning down, and *argeō* meaning "to be idle"). You could say it means to be in neutral, to idle down, or to put into neutral. It doesn't seem to mean to "destroy" as the KJV says or even to *"be done away with"* as the NASB says, but rather to "disengage." *Katargeō* is the word used in 1 Corinthians 13 with the *"gifts of prophecy"* and with the *"gifts of knowledge."* Sin's power is broken, and in that sense, destroyed, or done away with when it is shifted into neutral by our Lord Jesus, who conquered it, by coming to live in us. But, it still has the potential in our lives when we choose not to live surrendered to Christ. It hasn't ceased to exist. Read Colossians 2:6 and write it below.

_____

_____

_____

> *How did you receive Christ? By faith! Bowed, repentant, and surrendered before Him knowing that you could not save yourself.*

How did you receive Christ? By faith! Bowed, repentant, and surrendered before Him knowing that you could not save yourself. Understanding this, then what do you think Colossians 2:6 telling us?

_____

_____

_____

DAILY REFLECTION

As a believer, do you still struggle with sin? (You can be honest here!) You are a believer, but you still struggle with sin. Take a moment and think about the things you struggle with as a believer. It is important to realize that when you become a Christian, you stop chasing after sin and sin starts chasing after you! There is a big difference. So far we have learned that we are under grace and are set free from the dominion of sin! But, even though we have this newfound freedom from sin's domination, we will always struggle with the tendencies of the flesh. Think about what you have learned in Romans as it relates to this dilemma. What have you learned that can specifically help you daily as you battle with the flesh and the temptation to let it be master over you? How can we render it what it already is, powerless?

_____

_____

_____

_____

_____

DAY 4

WE ARE FREED FROM SIN

Let's read Romans 6:7–11 and focus in on the word "freed." The word in the Greek is *dikaióō*, meaning to declare righteous or to show to be righteous. We have been declared righteous if we have died with Christ in salvation, but we have also been shown to be righteous. Think about your life. Is there any evidence that you have been shown to be righteous?

_____

_____

_____

WORD STUDY
"Freed"

The Greek word translated "freed" in Romans 6:7 is *Dikaióō*, which is translated "justified" in Romans 5:1. (See Day One on "justification.")

Paul goes on to say in verse 8, *"now if we have died with Christ, we believe that we shall also live with Him."* The word "with" here comes from the word *sun*, the same word we studied in verse 5. What does it mean in this verse?

_____

_____

_____

Belief must affect our behavior or it isn't true Belief.

The word "believe" here is in the present tense. We "are believing." Belief must affect our behavior or it is not belief. What is affecting the way you live day by day?

_____

". . . That we shall also live with Him." When would this be? Obviously, we will live with Him in Glory! But, is that what Paul is referring to in this verse? Isn't he saying that each day when we get up, we get up with the fact that we cannot be separated from Christ, which totally affects the way we live?

"Knowing that Christ, having been raised from the dead, is never to die again; death no longer is master over Him. For the death that He died, He died to sin, once for all; but the life that He lives, He lives to God." (verses 9–10)

Where does Christ live now?

_____

_____

_____

Turn to Galatians 2:20. What does this tell you about where Christ lives?

_____

_____

Now, if He lives in us, the life He lives is pulling us towards God, right? Turn to Romans 5:10 and write this verse below.

_____

> _His death and resurrection saved us from the penalty of sin, but He has come to live in us to save us from the power of sin!_

It is not His death that saves us from the power of sin, but His life! His death and resurrection saves us from the penalty of sin, but He has come to live in us to save us from the power of sin! He has given us His life. He has, with His life; given us then a prejudiced will over sin.

"Even so, consider yourselves to be dead to sin, but alive to God in Christ Jesus" (verse 11). The word _"consider"_ in the original Greek is _logizomai,_ meaning "to come to a conclusion about something." It means to reason something out to its conclusion. This word is translated _"reckon"_ in the KJV. We are dead to the sin, its penalty and its power, but to contrast that, we are ALIVE to God in Christ Jesus!

DAILY REFLECTION

Well friend, we've almost completed yet another week. Are you starting to grasp that you are not only dead to sin, but you are ALIVE IN CHRIST? Do you live in the abundant life He has promised to give you? Jesus so desires to live His abundant life through you.

Pray right now that He will make Himself known to you and teach you to live in the glorious abundant life He longs to give to you.

DAY FIVE

NOW WHAT?

Today is our last day for this lesson. Let's jump right in and look at verse 12 of Romans 6. *"Therefore do not let sin reign in your mortal body that you obey its lusts."*

The Greek verb used here for "do not let sin reign" is a present imperative active. The imperative is a command. Is there an option here? Based on this verse, what do you need to do about sin in your life?

According to verse 12, what kind of body do we all have?

Read verse 6. What kind of body is mentioned in this verse?

There is a problem with this sinful, mortal body. *"Therefore do not let sin reign in your mortal body that you obey its _____."*

What are these lusts? The plural form of the Greek word translated "lusts" is *epithumia*. *Epi* is an intensifier and the word *thumia* is the word for passion. The idea is something that our flesh desires intensely; it compels us.

Look at James 1:13–15 and write what you learn from these verses.

How do we make certain that these lusts are not obeyed? Read Romans 6:13 and write it below.

According to this verse, what were the Roman believers doing with their bodies?

They were presenting their bodies to sin! The word "presenting" is in the present active tense. Interesting isn't it? They were believers, but they were presently and actively presenting their bodies to sin. What are the "members" of your body?

Look at Romans 6:19 and Romans 12:4, write what you learn from these verses.

The word for *"present"* is the word *paristemi*, meaning "to place beside." Paul is basically trying to say, "Don't get near it!" What is the opposite of placing your body and its members alongside that which is unrighteousness?

Victory is not me overcoming sin; it's Jesus overcoming me!

DAILY REFLECTION

The way you stop presenting your body to unrighteousness is to present it to righteousness. It is not what you turn away from, but what you turn to! Remember Romans 6:14, *"For sin shall not be master over you, for you are not under law, but under grace."* Is sin mastering your life? What are you presenting yourself to? Victory is not you overcoming sin; it's Jesus overcoming you! Take some time now to reflect on what you have learned this week. Write what God has taught you. It's always good to write it out because it helps you remember and process what God is saying.

LESSON 3

THE FRUSTRATION OF TRYING TO LIVE UNDER THE LAW

We have seen that we have been set free from the "performance mentality" of the Law. We are now under the enabling power of Grace. We are never to think that the demands of God have been withdrawn, but we are to realize that God now lives in us in the person of His Holy Spirit to produce what His law enables. But there are those times when we choose to put ourselves back under law. We like rules; we like formulas; we like the personal benefit of doing things ourselves. Why? Because we like ourselves! We like to glory in what we can do for God. But, the problem is that the law condemns our human righteousness. God is not impressed. Why would He live in us if we could do it ourselves? For those of us who enjoy doing it ourselves, trying to do what God says we must do in our own power is the guarantee for frustration in our lives like we have never known before. Let's look at chapter 7 of Romans.

> *"We like rules; we like formulas; we like the personal benefit*
> *of doing things ourselves."*

DAY 1

BEARING FRUIT UNTO DEATH

Read through Romans chapter 7. What impression did you get as you read through this concerning the law?

_____

_____

_____

Paul is concerned about a person seeking to live *"under the law"* in chapter 7. The word "law" is used 77 times in the entire book of Romans. How many times is it used in chapter 7?

_____

What main concept Paul is pointing out in verse 1?

_____

_____

The definite article in the Greek always identifies something specific. The definite article is not used in this phrase in verse 1, *"or do you not know, brethren (for I am speaking to those who know the law)."* He is speaking here of those who know "law," or those who know how "law" works. This could be any law including the Ten Commandments. Paul goes on to say, *"that the law has jurisdiction over a person as long as he lives."* Whatever law you want to talk about, that law has jurisdiction over a person as long as he lives! So, "living" is being under law. As long as a person is alive, he is under law.

What illustration does Paul give in verse 2?

_____

_____

_____

How is the "married woman" freed from her husband?

_____

_____

Isn't it the _____ of her husband?

Now, I know this is getting deep, but stay with me and remember to keep the main idea the main idea! According to verse 3, she can't be married to _____ husbands at once. The first husband must _____ for her to be free to marry another. In order for her to be free, there must be a death!

Do you see what Paul is doing? He goes on in verse 4 to say, *"Therefore my brethren, you also were made to die to the Law through the body of Christ, that you might be joined to another, to Him who was raised from the dead, that we might bear fruit for God."*

When did we die?

_____

_____

_____

Read again Romans 6:1–5. We were once "under" the law, but now in Christ, we are under grace!

> *Romans 6:1–5 says in essence that though we were once under the*
> *Law, through Christ, we are now under grace!*

DAILY REFLECTION

When we now relate to Christ through surrender, we bear fruit for righteousness! Romans 7:4. Now, look at verse 5. To what end was the fruit destined when we lived under law?

_____

_____

We once lived under the controlling, condemning power of the law and the result, no matter how religious or good it looked, was fruit unto death. It would not last. I have always said that when you squeeze a fruit, what's on the inside will come out! What kind of fruit are you bearing my friend? If you are experiencing the frustration of living under the law, you are bearing fruit unto death. All of your "good works" are dead in the sight of God. But if you are living under grace, you will be bearing fruit unto righteousness! Let God do a fruit inspection on you right now. Search your heart, and allow Him to get rid of the bad fruit, and in prayer trust Him to produce the kind of fruit in you, which yields righteousness.

DAY 2

FREED FROM THE LAW

Now, according to Romans 7:6, what is our new position to the law?

_____

_____

_____

The word "released" comes from the Greek word *katargeo*, which we saw in Romans 6:6. *Katargeo* presents the idea of something being rendered inactive or idle. The Law still exists, but its hold on us has been released. Christ fulfilled the Law as a man, the God man, and now lives in us to enable what the Law demands. The word *"bound"* implies that we were held fast to the Law. The Greek word from which the word "bound" is translated is in the imperfect passive tense. Imperfect means that our being bound was a continuous condition, and the passive voice suggests that we didn't initiate it. The term *"oldness of the letter"* refers to our obedience and bondage to the letter of the Law, the type of obedience which the Law demands.

Read Romans 7:6 again and note that we now serve in the _____ of the _____. The word "newness" relates to an entirely new way to live. The newness now enables us to be what God demands that we be.

According to verse 7, which reads, *"what shall we say then? Is the Law sin? May it never be! On the contrary, I would not have come to know sin except through the Law; for I would not have known about coveting if the Law had not said, 'You shall not covet.'"*

> *"What shall we say then? Is the Law sin? May it never be!"*
>
> Romans 7:7a

How would we ever know we are sinners without the law?

In fact, the law is a good thing! Also, according to verse 8, which reads, *"But sin, taking opportunity through the commandment, produced in me coveting of every kind; for apart from the Law sin is dead."*

What was it that actually aroused sin?

The Greek word translated "opportunity" in this verse literally means, "to build a base camp" like the military would do when invading a land. Paul goes on to say in verse 8, "For _____ from the _____ sin is _____ ."

Wow! Write any thoughts on this you may have so far.

_____

_____

_____

_____

DAILY REFLECTION

Now, according to Romans, Paul has mentioned two different ways that sin is manifested. We looked at these two ways a little bit last week. One, in Romans 1:18–32 is rebellion. The other, in Romans 2:1–3:20 is religion. How does your flesh tend to react to law? Do you rebel? Or, do you pride yourself in the way that you do everything right while at the same time very condemning of others who are not as "spiritual" as you think you are. Think through this and write your answer below.

_____

_____

_____

_____

We all have our fleshly patterns. Pray and ask God to help you surrender to Him in every way. Although we will never lose these patterns until we get to heaven, God can give us the strength through His grace and our surrender to allow Him to control us when our flesh would fight to do otherwise.

DAY THREE:

MEN OF FLESH

Now we come to the most controversial part of Romans chapter 7—one that has separated Christian friends and ministries and caused quite a stir. The question comes up, is Paul writing about a time when he was lost, or is he speaking of another lost person? Remember, the subject of chapter 7 is the Law. Whether we are living under it or not, the results of living under the Law are the same if you are lost or if you are saved.

Let's dissect verse 14. *"For we know that the Law is spiritual; but I am of flesh, sold into bondage to sin."* The Greek word translated "spiritual" is the word *pneumatikos*. It means "spiritual in and out," totally of the Spirit. First Corinthians 2:14 says, *"But a natural man does not accept the things of the Spirit of God; for they are foolishness to him, and he cannot understand them, because they are spiritually appraised."* The Greek word for "natural" is the word *psuchikos*. It is used here and as an adjective in James 3:15: *"This wisdom is not that which comes down from above, but is earthly, natural [psuchikos], demonic."* It is also used as an adjective in Jude 1:19, *"These are the ones who cause divisions, worldly-minded [psuchikos], devoid of the Spirit."* It is not used to speak of a believer, but rather of an unbeliever.

The word translated "flesh," *sarkikos*, as mentioned above in Romans 7:14 is also used in 1 Corinthians 3:1, *"And I, brethren, could not speak to you as to spiritual men, but as to men of flesh, as to babes in Christ."* The part to focus on is the phrase *"men of flesh."* Is Paul speaking of believers here? Yes! We see that the word *sarkikos* can be used to speak of believers. Based on this, what are your thoughts on whether or not Paul was lost or saved when he wrote Romans 7?

_____

_____

_____

I believe Paul was saved. There was something about Paul that was definitely lured to sin and that was aroused by the law. It was his flesh! This is the struggle as we saw earlier that even though we are freed from the dominion of sin, we have to be careful to not let sin be master over us.

Now, what are some of the frustrations of living under law? Romans 7:15 says, *"For that which I am doing, I do not understand; for I am not practicing what I would like to do, but I am doing the very thing I hate."* Have you ever felt this way? Explain a recent occurrence of that.

_____

_____

_____

_____

Paul goes on to say in verse 16, *"But if I do the very thing I do not wish to do, I agree with the Law, confessing that it is good."* How is Paul tying this in with what he has already said? The law is _____ .

Lastly, in verse 17, Paul says, *"So now, no longer am I the one doing it, but sin which indwells me."*

Does an unbeliever have a "no longer am I the one doing it" excuse? So, is this person saved or lost?

_____

DAILY REFLECTION

Well, that is a difficult passage to get through. I hope that you were blessed as you saw the meaning come to life by looking at what Paul was saying in the Greek language. We can all relate with Paul in Romans 7, can't we? Living the Christian life can be such a struggle when we try to live it in our own strength. Describe what your life is like when you seek to do things in your own strength, trying to accomplish what only God can do in your life.

_____

_____

_____

_____

DAY 4

NOTHING GOOD DWELLS IN MY FLESH

Isn't it fun to live in your own strength, under the Law, seeking to do for God rather than allowing Him to do through you? This statement sounds ridiculous after what we have learned this week; but the sad truth is that many of us continue to choose to live this way, all the while as miserable as can be. Let's continue to look in Romans 7, as Paul continues to stress the wickedness of that old flesh.

Romans 7:18 says, *"For I know that nothing good dwells in me, that is, in my flesh; for the wishing is present in me, but the doing of the good is not."*

Paul says that _____ good dwells in him. But, notice his reference point, *"that is, in my _____."*

The term "flesh" is used two ways in Romans.

First, as literal flesh and blood. One example of this usage is in Romans 1:3, *"concerning His Son, who was born of a descendant of David according to the flesh."*

Secondly, as an attitude of "doing it our way." You can see this in Romans 7:5, *"For while we were in the flesh, the sinful passions, which were aroused by the Law, were at work in the members of our body to bear fruit for death."*

There is no coincidence that the word is used in reference to the body of flesh and to the mindset of evil that is resident in it. There is nothing "good" in the flesh. Its attitude of pleasing oneself hinders us from doing what the Spirit demands. *"For the good that I wish, I do not do; but I practice the very evil that I do not wish"* (Romans 7:19).

Now read verse 20. Paul repeats what he said back in verse 17. Write it out in your own words.

_____

_____

_____

Paul has made a discovery. The greatest preacher of grace in the New Testament has made a discovery! Read verse 21 and write it below.

_____

_____

_____

Do you see it? *"I find then the principle that evil is present in me, the one who wishes to do good."* Paul realized that though he was now in Christ and under grace, evil was still present within his flesh.

> *The flesh, apart from Christ's intervention, is a hater of God and*
> *an enemy of the cross.*

DAILY REFLECTION

Do you realize the wickedness of your flesh? Until you do, you will never realize your need for God's enabling power in our lives. As much as we feel like we love the Lord, it's hard to understand that the flesh, apart from Christ's intervention, is a hater of God and an enemy of the cross. Pray and ask God to let you see yourself as you really are without Him. It is a humbling experience, but oh the joy when you then see yourself as God sees you through the blood of Christ. Take some time and meditate on what you have learned.

_____

_____

_____

_____

_____

_____

DAY FIVE:

THE DESIRE OF YOUR HEART

Let's start today by reviewing what we have learned so far this week. Take some time to recall what God has taught you about being under the Law.

_____

_____

Now, let's look at the heart of Paul and his desires to do what God wanted. Verse 22 says, *"For I joyfully concur with the law of God in the inner man."* This term "inner man" is used here and in Ephesians 3:16, *"that He would grant you, according to the riches of His glory, to be strengthened with power through His Spirit in the inner man."* Paul equates this term with the heart in the next verse in Ephesians.

This term is also used to contrast the outer man in 2 Corinthians 4:16: *"Therefore we do not lose heart, but though our outer man is decaying, yet our inner man is being renewed day by day."* Here Paul uses the term "inner man" to describe the heart of hearts, where the Spirit of God dwells. It is Paul's desire in his heart of hearts that he concurs with God's law.

But, Paul has noticed something different that is totally against his inner desire to please God. Write verse 23.

_____

_____

_____

Notice the phrase *"in the members of my body."* What kind of body? (Romans 6:6)

_____

_____

_____

Have you ever awakened in the morning with nothing but the desire to please God, and by the end of the day you were saying what is said in verse 24, *"Wretched man that I am! Who will set me free from the body of this death!"*? Write out the last time this happened to you.

_____

_____

_____

Notice that Paul didn't say "what" shall deliver me, but _____ shall deliver me!

"Thanks be to God through Jesus Christ our Lord! So then, on the one hand I myself with my mind am serving the law of God, but on the other, with my flesh the law of sin" (Romans 7:25). It is always true that when we do things our way as believers, we are serving the

_____ .

What is the first thing one does when he or she fails God on a consistent basis? Doubts his salvation! Have you ever done that? When?

_____

_____

_____

_____

_____

What is the answer? It is found in Romans 8:1, *"There is therefore now no condemnation for those who are in Christ Jesus."* What do these words mean to you? Do they comfort you? How?

_____

_____

_____

_____

_____

"For the law of the Spirit of life in Christ Jesus has set you free from the law of sin and death" (Romans 8:2).

The word "law" can mean "principle." What principle do we live under as believers? We live under the authority of the Holy Spirit of God now. He is the One and only that bestows life in us and manifests it through us.

Romans 8:3 goes on to say, *"For what the Law could not do, weak as it was through the flesh, God did: sending His own Son in the likeness of sinful flesh and as an offering for sin, He condemned sin in the flesh."*

> "As it is written, 'There is none righteous, not even one; There is none who understands, There is none who seeks for God.'"
>
> Romans 3:11

Man could not fulfill the law. But, God did by sending His Son Jesus Christ, the God man, to fulfill the law for us. In doing so, He condemned sin (rebellious and religious) **in the flesh!**

Why? Verse 4 says, *"In order that the requirement of the Law might be fulfilled in us, who do not walk according to the flesh, but according to the Spirit."*

Well Friend! We have finished another week. Isn't the Scripture full of wisdom? Do you feel a load lifted off of you as you study? I know there are many times full of discouragement, failure, and even doubting your very salvation. Remember that there is now no condemnation for those who are in Christ Jesus! We have been set free. What is your heart's desire? You may not be where you want to be in your walk with the Lord, but in your heart of hearts, if you cry out to Him as Abba Father, He hears you! He is mindful that we are but dust, as the psalmist so accurately put it. He knows our weakness, but above all, He knows our hearts. (See I John 3:20.)

LESSON 4

RECEIVING WHAT IS ALREADY OURS

I was preaching at a church in the South, and when I returned to the hotel after the service, I noticed that one of the parking places appeared to have a spot on the pavement that was blackened or burned. The friend driving me to the hotel told me about a business owner who was in town for a convention. Of course, his company paid all of his expenses. He came in one night and was drunk out of his mind. Walking up to the registration desk of his hotel he asked, "How much is a room?" The clerk told him, and the man cursed and said, "I wouldn't pay that to stay here!" He was so drunk he didn't realize the room was already paid for. He left the lobby and went to his car, which was parked out front. There he decided in his drunken stupor to sleep it off in his car. He lit a cigarette and slowly fell asleep. The cigarette fell onto his shirt, setting it on fire and consequently the rest of his clothes. The car and the man burned to death just a few yards away from what was his and already paid for. He was too drunk to realize what he already had.

> *"Many Christians do not realize that the Christian life is not a matter of "getting something" once we have Christ, but receiving what we already have in Him."*

In a similar way, many Christians do not realize what is theirs in Christ. They do not understand that the Christian life is not a matter of "getting something" once we have Christ, but receiving what we already have in Him. We plead and beg for what we already have but do not realize it. Well, this lesson, centered on the prayer Paul prays at the end of Ephesians 3, will hopefully help us understand what is already ours in Christ.

DAY 1:

A DWELLING PLACE OF GOD

Read Paul's prayer in Ephesians 3:14–21. Paul says in verse 14, "For this reason I bow my knees. . . ." What reason could he be talking about? Normally to find the answer to a question like this you would just back up a few verses to discover it. But look at verse 1 of chapter 3 and write it below.

Note that Paul starts verse 14 in the same way. I believe that he begins his prayer in verse 1, but doesn't pick it back up until verse 14. If that is the case, then we will have to back up to chapter 2 to discover the reason Paul bows his knees to the Father.

Read Ephesians 2:19–22. As Paul sums up his thoughts, notice verse 22, "in whom you also are being built together into a dwelling of God in the Spirit." Now, Paul is a converted Jew writing to converted Gentiles. He says to them that they are *being built together into a dwelling of God in the Spirit."* A dwelling of God. Wow!

If you are a believer, do you realize that God lives in you? Now, think about that for a minute. God lives in you! We looked at that a little in Romans 6. All that you need to be, all that He wants you to be, you already have in Him who lives within you!

Paul says in Ephesians 3:16, "that He would grant you, according to the riches of His glory, to be strengthened with power through His Spirit in the inner man." The word translated "according" is the Greek word *kata*. Some translations say "out of" instead of "according" but I believe the Greek word *ek*, meaning "out of," would have been used instead of *kata*. But *kata* is used, so it conveys the idea of God strengthening us according to the riches of His glory. When "according to" is used, it reflects the measure from which we are being strengthened.

Speaking of the "riches of His glory," now you could say that the "riches of His glory" is the warehouse of supply that we are to draw strength from. What is in that storehouse? Read Ephesians 3:8 and write it below.

_____

_____

_____

What kind of riches? _____

The word "unfathomable" means "unsearchable." Now, we are to be strengthened by the measure of the unsearchable riches of Christ! Isn't that a marvelous thought?

> *"Seeing that His divine power has granted us everything pertaining to life and godliness, through the true knowledge of Him who called us by His own glory and excellence."*
>
> 2 Peter 1:3

In Ephesians 1:18 Paul says, "I pray that the eyes of your heart may be enlightened, so that you may know what is the hope of His calling, what are the riches of the glory of His inheritance in the saints."

Where are our riches? _____

Where is Christ? _____

It is _____ inheritance which is _____ us.

He lives in _____ .

DAILY REFLECTION

Is there anything that you need to live the Christian life that you don't already have in Christ? Isn't it wonderful that all we need we have in Christ who lives in us? You don't have to spend your life trying to attain righteous living to somehow please God. Instead, realize that YOU are God's dwelling place through His Holy Spirit and because of that you are righteous in God's sight. Pray and ask God to help you live in the light of this truth. Christ IS your righteousness and longs to live His life in and through you as you are surrendered to Him. Write out your thoughts in response to Him now.

DAY 2

UNSEARCHABLE RICHES

Now, today we are going to begin to look at some of those "unsearchable riches" that we have in Christ. Look at Ephesians 1:3. "Blessed be the God and Father of our Lord Jesus Christ, who has blessed us with every spiritual blessing in the heavenly places in Christ."

Are there any spiritual blessings left out here? Paul says we have all spiritual blessing!

Again, where are these blessings? _____

_____

Wait a minute. "I'm confused", you say. "I thought Christ lived in me! Here it says He '*is in the Heavenly places.*'" Well, let's make certain we understand this. Christ is at the right hand of the Father. But, He lives in us through the Person of His Spirit.

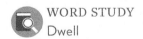

WORD STUDY
Dwell

In Romans 8:11, Paul describes the Holy Spirit dwelling in us (*"But if the Spirit . . . dwells in you. . . ."*). The Greek word translated "dwells" here is *oikeō*, which conveys the idea of occupying a house, home, or dwelling, which in biblical times could have been describing a tent. Remember we learned that Paul says in Ephesians 2:22, that as Christians we are *"being built together into a dwelling of God in the Spirit."* The word "dwelling" in this verse is translated from *katoikētērion*, a noun related to the verb *oikeo* that simply means dwelling place or home.

Romans 8:11 says, *"But if the Spirit of Him who raised Jesus from the dead dwells in you, He who raised Christ Jesus from the dead will also give life to your mortal bodies through His Spirit who indwells you."*

Who is the subject here? _____

It is "He who raised Jesus from the dead." Whose Spirit is this? It is the Spirit of God who dwells in us.

1 John 4:12–13 says, *"No one has beheld God at any time; if we love one another, God abides in us, and His love is perfected in us. By this we know that we abide in Him, and He in us, because He has given us of His Spirit."*

His Spirit abides in us. He has given us of His Spirit.

Second Corinthians 3:17–18 says, *"Now the Lord is the Spirit; and where the Spirit of the Lord is, there is liberty. But we all, with unveiled face beholding as in a mirror the glory of the Lord, are being transformed into the same image from glory to glory, just as from the Lord, the Spirit."*

Who is "the Lord" in this context? _____

_____

Read Romans 8:9 and write it below.

_____

_____

_____

_____

The Holy Spirit is called the Spirit of Christ. So, the Holy Spirit and Christ are one. There are not three gods, but one God in three persons.

John 14:23 says, *"Jesus answered and said unto him, 'If anyone loves Me, he will keep My word; and My Father will love him, and we will come to him, and make our abode with him.'"*

The word for "abode" refers to a place where one dwells. When He says, "We will come to him", who does the word "we" refer to?

_____

_____

_____

We must realize that the Holy Spirit IS God. He is the Spirit of the Father and the Spirit of Christ. He lives in us! Now, all of our blessings are in Christ, who lives in us!

Look at Ephesians 1:3 again and write it below.

_____

_____

_____

_____

DAILY REFLECTION

Well friend, we have EVERY spiritual blessing in Christ. Colossians 1:27 says, *"God willed to make known (to His saints) what is the riches of the glory of this mystery among the Gentiles, which is Christ in you, the hope of glory."* Where are these unsearchable riches found? In Christ! And Christ dwells within you through the person of His Holy Spirit. Take some time now to meditate on this incredible truth and write down your thoughts in thanksgiving to God.

_____

_____

_____

_____

_____

_____

_____

DAY 3

EVERY SPIRITUAL BLESSING IS OURS IN CHRIST JESUS

Now, let's focus on the blessings we have in Christ. Ephesians 1:1 says, *"Paul, an apostle of Christ Jesus by the will of God, to the saints who are at Ephesus, and who are faithful in Christ Jesus."*

The Greek word for "saints" here is *hagios*. We will not exhaust the meaning of the word in this study, but the word in its root meaning is "to be set apart." A Saint is one who has been "set apart" in Christ. We are "set apart" unto Him to use as He wills. We are His vessels with an eternal purpose of serving Him.

With this in mind, as a saint, what is our first and only purpose in life?

_____

_____

_____

If our purpose is to be used as He wills, since we are set apart unto Him, then who has total authority over our lives? Keeping this in mind, write out what this means to your life.

_____

_____

_____

_____

One of the "riches" or blessings that we are to be strengthened by is that we are "set apart" for His purposes. We have a divine purpose in our life. Verse 4 says, *"just as He chose us in Him before the foundation of the world, that we should be holy and blameless before Him."*

He chose us in Him! The word "chose" originates from the Greek word *eklegō*. *Eklegō* actually comes from two Greek words; *ek* meaning "out of" and *lego* which means "to say, to select, or to call." He called us out; He selected us.

Now, there is much controversy over this very important subject, and we are not going to attempt to solve it in this study. But here is one question we can answer. Did you find Him or did He find you?

_____

_____

_____

What does that say to you today while you are doing this study?

_____

_____

_____

Are you special to Him?_____

Do you feel special? _____

If you don't feel special, does that change what His Word says?

_____

_____

With all the rejection in this world, what does this passage in Ephesians 1:4 say to you?

_____

_____

Ephesians 1:5 says, *"He predestined us to adoption as sons through Jesus Christ to Himself, according to the kind intention of His will."* The word "predestined" is our English equivalent of the Greek *proorizō*. *Proorizō* refers to the purpose God has for those who are "called out or selected." What is that purpose?

_____

_____

_____

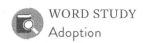

WORD STUDY
Adoption

Huiothesía ("adoption") is a technical term used only by Paul five times (Rom. 8:15, 23; 9:4; Gal. 4:5; Eph. 1:5). Paul in these passages is alluding to a Greek and Roman custom rather than a Hebrew one. Since *huiothesia* was a technical term in Roman law for an act that had specific legal and social effects, there is much probability that Paul had some reference to that in his use of the word. Adoption, when thus legally performed, put a man in every respect in the position of a son by birth to him who had adopted him, so that he possessed the same rights and owed the same obligations. (*The Complete Word Study Dictionary* [Strong's #5206])

The word for *"adoption as sons"* is the word *huiothesia. Huiothesia* is based on two words: *huios,* meaning "mature sons" and *tithemi,* meaning "to place, or to set, or to assign or to purpose." God's purpose for us is to be His "mature sons." When will that purpose be completed? Read Romans 8:23.

This purpose will be complete at the redemption of our bodies! In other words, when our bodies are redeemed or delivered from their present state into glorified bodies. God "predestined" that this will take place one day. What does this say to you?

_____

_____

_____

How can you be strengthened by this truth?

_____

_____

_____

Redemption through His blood is another spiritual blessing we have in Him. Read Ephesians 1:7 and write it below.

_____

_____

_____

The Greek word *apolutrosis* is translated "redemption" in this verse. *Apolutrosis* comes from *apo,* meaning "away from" and *lutrosis,* meaning "to purchase." *Apolutrosis* conveys the idea of God purchasing us away from the slave block of sin. God has indeed purchased us away from sin's power and penalty. What was the price God had to pay? *"In Him, we have redemption through His blood."*

Earlier in our study we talked about how even though we are freed from the dominion of sin, we still struggle with our flesh and sin being master over us. What problem of sin do you struggle with?

_____

_____

_____

_____

What do these verses tell you that can help you when you are tempted by sin's power?

_____

_____

_____

_____

Do you have to say "yes" to its lure? _____

Why not?

_____

_____

_____

Another blessing we have in Christ is the forgiveness of sins. Looking back into verse 7, the word "forgiveness" is translated from the Greek *aphesis*. It means "to release from bondage or imprisonment." What does this say to you? Have you been living under the lie that you have to do what the flesh says? What does this tell you that contradicts that lifestyle? Take a moment and meditate on these questions.

_____

_____

_____

_____

Paul says in verse 13, *"In Him, you also, after listening to the message of truth, the gospel of your salvation—having also believed, you were sealed in Him with the Holy Spirit of promise."*

What had to happen before you trusted Christ? You had to "listen to the message of truth." Now, once you heard the Word of Truth and you believed, what happened?

_____

_____

_____

_____

_____

The Greek word *sphragizo*, translated in this verse as "sealed," means "to put a mark on someone or something, causing it to be authentic." It's kind of like a brand. What is the "mark" that God put on us?

_____

_____

We are branded for Christ, like the cattle are branded and
everywhere they go, people know whose they are. Do we live in such
a way as "set apart" that others know who we belong to?

The mark is His Holy Spirit! How long does the Holy Spirit take up residence in us as God's mark? Read Ephesians 4:30 to answer this question.

_____

_____

_____

My Friend, you are sealed in Him until the final day of redemption, the day you get a glorified body.

DAILY REFLECTION

Wow! We are blessed with so many spiritual blessings in Christ. Just from studying this one passage in Ephesians, do you see how "rich" you are in Christ? God chose us before the foundation of the world and granted us adoption as sons of God! He redeems us and forgives us of sins, and seals us forever by His precious Holy Spirit who lives within us. Pray and ask God to help you realize what you have in Christ. Write out your thoughts of how each of these truths can strengthen you today.

_____

_____

_____

_____

_____

_____

_____

_____

_____

DAY 4

FAR ABOVE ALL POWER AND DOMINION

You know, a lot of people are getting sidetracked in their Christian walk by going around and chasing demons and have lost their focus of the power of the One who lives within them! Although Satan and his forces are powerful and we should not take that for granted, let's look in the Word and see if that is what we are to focus upon.

Ephesians 1:18–23 says, *"I pray that the eyes of your heart may be enlightened, so that you may know what is the hope of His calling, what are the riches of the glory of His inheritance in the saints, and what is the surpassing greatness of His power toward us who believe. These are in accordance with the working of the strength of His might which He brought about in Christ, when He raised Him from the dead, and seated Him at His right hand in the heavenly places, far above all rule and authority and power and dominion, and every name that is named, not only in this age, but also in the one to come. And He put all things in subjection under His feet, and gave Him as head over all things to the church, which is His body, the fullness of Him who fills all in all."*

Note in verse 19 that the *"greatness of His power"* is directed toward us.

Now, what kind of power does Paul speak of (verse 20)?

_____

_____

Resurrection power! Look up Philippians 3:10 and write how this verse relates to what we are discussing.

_____

_____

_____

Back in our passage in Ephesians, where is Jesus seated?

"Far above" what? _____

Do the devil and his demons fit this criterion?

_____

_____

_____

Note verse 21 of our text. *"Far above all rule and authority and power and dominion. . . ."* Does "all" mean all? So then, what does this tell you about Jesus' power over Satan?

_____

_____

_____

The words "far above" are translated from two Greek words, *huper*, meaning "above" and *ano*, meaning "up or above." You could say that Jesus' power is "above" and then even higher "above." My interpretation is "out of sight!" Put the devil and his demons up next to Christ, and they would not show up on the scale.

DAILY REFLECTION

*Remember that anything that would ever come to us
from the devil has to go by God first.*

Now, how much sense does it make to focus on something that doesn't even compare to Christ and to who He is? What is your focus? Remember, our flesh is usually our own worst enemy and anything that would ever come to us from the devil has to go by God first. I like to think of it as being filtered through His loving hands to ultimately bring good out of it in our lives. The Word says that ALL things are "from Him, through Him, and to Him" (Romans 11:36). Don't let yourself get distracted by the power of Satan. It's a very popular subject in our day and time. Put all that aside, and allow Christ to fill your heart and mind with His ability and His power as being far above all else. Take some time to write out your thoughts.

_____

_____

_____

_____

_____

_____

_____

_____

_____

_____

_____

DAY 5

STRENGTHENED IN THE INNER MAN

Well, as I said before, there is no way we can exhaust all of the riches that are ours in Christ Jesus! They truly are "unsearchable"! But, back in Ephesians 3:16 we read, *"that He would grant you, according to the riches of His glory, to be strengthened with power through His Spirit in the inner man."*

The word "strengthen" is the word meaning "proven strength" or "dominion." Paul is praying that they would have "dominion" or be proven to be strong over those things that can so easily cause them to fail. It is according to the riches of His glory that we are "proven strong." Not in ourselves!

The Greek word translated "power" in Ephesians 3:16 is *dunamis*, which means "the ability to do what must be done." The source of this power is through His <u>Spirit</u>.

Now, where does the Spirit live? Look back at the text, *"in the <u>inner</u> man."*

Where is the inner man? Verse 17 says, "so that Christ may dwell in your hearts." The "heart" and the "inner man" are the same. The Spirit talked about here is the Spirit of Christ! Christ lives in us through the person of the Holy Spirit, in our hearts.

So, does the strengthening come from within or from without? It comes from within, because Christ dwells within our hearts. All the religions of the world are external, from the outside in. But, Christianity is not a religion! It is a relationship and begins from within instead of from without! Our strengthening begins on the <u>inside</u> before it ever shows up on the outside.

> *"Now to Him who is able to do far more abundantly beyond all*
> *that we ask or think, according to the power that works within us,*
> *to Him be the glory in the church and in Christ Jesus to all*
> *generations forever and ever. Amen."*

Ephesians 3:20, 21

DAILY REFLECTION

What a week of study we have had! Has God helped you to realize what you have in Him? What about your strength, are you trying to get it from outside sources instead of from the person of Jesus Christ? Have you fully realized that Christianity is not a religion, but a relationship? Take some time in prayer now. If you have never received Jesus Christ as your personal Savior, admit this to Him. Receive His forgiveness of sins and allow Him to seal you with His precious Holy Spirit. If you are His child, thank Him for the blessings and unsearchable riches that are yours because of His life in you! He not only gives you everything you need to live this Christian life, he also gives you strength in your inner man. It is His power that works it out in your life. Write out your thoughts or maybe a prayer to Him right now.

LESSON 5

APPROPRIATING WHAT WE HAVE IN CHRIST

"*Oh, the depth of the riches both of the wisdom and knowledge of God! How unsearchable are His judgments and unfathomable His ways! For who has known the mind of the LORD, or who became His counselor? Or who has first given to Him that it might be paid back to Him again? For from Him and through Him and to Him are all things. To Him be the glory forever. Amen.*" (Rom. 11:33-36)

My life will look different when I am appropriating these truths!
We are to learn to "accommodate" the Divine presence of God in our lives! We are to give Him full reign of our hearts.

How could anyone say it any better when they realize what God has done for us in Christ? We have seen so much of what we have in Him, but we have not even scratched the surface! His "riches" are "unsearchable." But the questions remain, "How do I appropriate what I have in Christ?" and, "What does my life look like when I am appropriating these truths?" This is what we will be looking at in this week's lesson.

DAY 1

MAKING CHRIST FEEL AT HOME IN YOUR HEART

Ephesians 3:17 says, "*so that Christ may dwell in your hearts through faith.*"

Now, the word "dwell" here is translated from the Greek word *katoikeo*. It comes from two Greek words, *kata* meaning "down," and oikeo, meaning "house or home." "Down home" for all you Southerners! This word doesn't mean to "indwell" because that took place already at salvation, as we have studied. Instead, it means to "be at home" in our hearts. What does it mean to not just be in someone's home, but to feel at home while you are there?

_____

_____

_____

We are to learn to "accommodate" the Divine presence of God in our lives! We are to give Him full reign of our hearts.

Let's think of the rooms that are in the house of the heart. First we have the room of our thoughts. Luke 9:47 says, *"But Jesus, knowing what they were thinking in their heart. . . ."* You might think this should say, "mind" instead of "heart." What does the mind have to do with the heart? Hebrews 4:12 says, *"For the Word of God is living and active and sharper than any two-edged sword, and piercing as far as the division of soul and spirit, of both joints and marrow and able to judge the thoughts and intentions of the heart."* You could say that the heart of our problem is the problem of our heart! It's not only a mind problem; it's a <u>heart</u> problem.

Are you making Christ ruler of the room of your thoughts? Look at Matthew 18:35, and write it below.

_____

_____

_____

Forgiveness is an attitude. Now we see a second room in our hearts. The room of our attitude. Forgiveness does not just sound forth from the lips, it must be settled in the heart. We confess to Him that we cannot forgive, and then He produces the forgiveness in our hearts. Who is it that you have not allowed Christ in your hearts to forgive? Look at John 14:1, "Let not your heart be troubled; believe in God, believe also in Me."

The word "troubled" comes from the Greek word *tarasso*, meaning to be "disturbed, frightened, or stirred up." It is a word that would define stress and is definitely an emotional word. Now we move into the room of our emotions. There are many rooms that we could name as rooms within our hearts, but for the sake of the study, we will focus on these three.

The room of our thoughts
The room of our attitudes
The room of our emotions

Look again at Ephesians 3:17 and write it below.

_____

_____

What is it that "accommodates" Christ in the rooms of our thoughts, attitudes, and emotions? Well, it says, *"Christ may dwell in your hearts through <u>faith</u>."*

What is faith?

_____

_____

_____

The word "faith" here is translated from the Greek word *pistis*. It comes from the word *pisteuo* and means to "believe." Both words derive from *peitho*, which means, "to be so fully persuaded by someone or something that you bow and surrender to it fully." It's faith that accommodates the divine presence of Christ in our hearts! When we trust Him and His Word to the point of obedience, then we are accommodating Him in the different rooms of our hearts. We are making Him feel at home in our hearts.

DAILY REFLECTION

Well, how are you doing in accommodating Christ in your heart? Remember, the heart of the problem is the problem of the heart! Think of the three rooms we have talked about. Are you surrendered to Him in your thoughts, your attitude, and your emotions? Christ wants you to recognize Him to be Lord of these areas in your heart. Christ has made His abode in us. Make Him comfortable today and give him the keys to the rooms of your heart. Examine your heart right now. Does Christ feel at home there? Until He does, He can never unleash His power in your life. Write down your thoughts below.

_____

_____

_____

_____

_____

_____

DAY 2

WHAT HAPPENS WHEN CHRIST IS AT HOME IN US

When Christ is accommodated, we will have surrendered to Him and His Word, and this will cause a change in our lifestyle that will be seen on the outside. Ephesians 4:1 says, *"I, therefore, the prisoner of the Lord, entreat you to walk in a manner worthy of the calling with which you have been called."*

What does Paul call himself in this verse?

_____

_____

He is in the same imprisonment that he was in when he wrote Philippians, Colossians, and Philemon. But, he is a not a prisoner of the Jews or the Romans, he is a "love slave" of Christ!

Do you realize that Christ IS your circumstance? Do you realize that when you are accommodating Him, no matter what the circumstance that surrounds you, you are His, and you have everything you need in Him?

The word "worthy" in Ephesians 4:1 is translated from the Greek word *axios*. It describes a set of scales that are balanced. If you put 100 pounds on one side of the scales, you have to put 100 pounds on the other side to balance it correctly. In Chapter 3, Paul has established one side of the scales. Now, in Chapter 4, he tells us how we can balance these scales by the way we live. One side of the scales is the "calling"; the other side is the "living" in a manner worthy of that calling. In short, Paul wants to match their walk with their talk.

When that happens, their lives will definitely be different, especially when they relate to others. Read Ephesians 4:2 and write it below.

_____

_____

_____

Paul lists some qualities here that will be present in our lives when we are accommodating Christ. Let's go through each one and find out what it means to us.

Humility – This is from the word *tapeinophrosune*. It comes from two words, *tapeinos* which means "to get as flat on the ground as you can because there is nothing about you that is worthy," and *phrosune*, which describes a particular mindset. Humility reflects the proper mindset one must have towards himself in light of who Christ is! Have you seen yourself in this light?

Gentleness – This is the word *prautes* in the Greek. It is used to describe meekness. Not weakness, but meekness! Like a horse that has been broken, all of its power has been put under control. It does not use its power for itself but for its master. Have you let Christ take over the reins of your heart in this manner? He wants to break us of our old ways and put a gentle spirit within us.

Patience – This word is *makrothumia* in the Greek. It means, "long suffering." *Makro* means "long," and *thumia* means "passionate suffering." Patience is the supernatural ability to put up with those in your life who are not loveable. Is Christ manifesting His ability to strengthen you in this area?

Forbearance – The word "forbearance" comes from the word *anecho* meaning "to hold up" or to "bear with." It comes from *ana* meaning "up", and *echo* meaning "to hold." You could say it means, "to hold each other up." When strife comes with a brother who is not being strengthened in the inner man by the power and presence of Christ, we then take the attitude of holding him up until he can get his feet back on the ground again. We do not split and run and cause further division! Think about how this is illustrated in your life, either positive or negative.

DAILY REFLECTION

What have you learned so far today about what your life is like when you are willing to accommodate the holy presence of Christ? Your life will be evidenced by these qualities on the outside when Christ is at home on the inside! Ask God to reveal Himself to you right now.

_____

_____

_____

_____

_____

_____

_____

_____

_____

DAY 3

DILIGENT TO PRESERVE THE UNITY OF THE SPIRIT

Ephesians 4:3 says, *"Being diligent to preserve the unity of the Spirit in the bond of peace."* There is only one word for "diligent" in the Greek text. The word is *spoudazō*, meaning "to make haste." It carries the idea of doing something with a sense of urgency. The phrase "to preserve" comes from *tereo*, meaning to guard like a watchman who is responsible to watch over a very important person. Think of it like the Secret Service agents and how diligent they are to protect the President.

Now, in the church, what is it that must be guarded with this same intensity? *"The unity of the Spirit"*! Wow. Am I saying that factions and conflicts in the church are something that must be prevented at all costs? Well, what do you think?

_____

_____

_____

_____

> *the peace of God is like a referee in our hearts*

Does your Bible say that we must be "diligent to 'produce' the unity of the Spirit"? If so, then throw it out and get you a proper translation! NO, it says we are to "preserve" that unity, not produce it. You can't preserve what you don't already have. God has already blessed us with the unity of the Spirit in Christ. We are "one" with one another in Him. Write out what this means to you in your relationships with others in your church. What is your responsibility to them?

_____

_____

_____

_____

How are we to preserve the unity of the Spirit?

_____

_____
_____
_____

"In the bond of peace." The word "peace" is a very important word. Look at Ephesians 1:2. What is the source of all peace?

_____
_____

Where does peace begin?

_____
_____
_____

Read Ephesians 2:14, 15, and 17. Who is our peace?

_____
_____
_____

This particular context of peace seems to be peace between the Gentile and the <u>Jew</u>—a very tall order for that time period. How does this speak to you today in your world?

_____
_____
_____

DAILY REFLECTION

One of the "weapons" we have in the warfare around us is found in Ephesians 6:15, *"and having shod your feet with the preparation of the gospel of peace."* Do you realize that if you are living in the "peace of God" which only comes when you have dealt with any conflicting deed or attitude in your life between you and God that this peace will overflow into your relationships with others? Is there anyone that you don't wish to be at peace with in your relationships?

_____
_____
_____

Whose forgiveness should you seek so that you can preserve the "unity of the Spirit"? Remember, being at peace with others starts by being at peace with God. Meditate on these truths now and ask God to reveal to you how He would have you to be diligent to preserve the unity in the Spirit.

_____

_____

_____

_____

_____

_____

_____

DAY 4

BEING AT PEACE WITH ALL MEN

Now, today I want you to take some time and just meditate on what we have learned so far. Get a separate sheet of paper and make a list of all the people that you have difficulty with—those who have offended you, or are just obnoxious in their attitude or behavior towards you. Now, realize that you cannot forgive them apart from God's grace working in your life. It is God that produces the forgiveness that He requires.

> *It is God that produces the forgiveness that He requires.*

If need be, and only if they are aware of your attitude towards them, pick up the telephone and call them and just ask for their forgiveness. I don't suggest calling or telling anyone about what they do not know when it comes to attitudes, etc. Doing this will many times only complicate the situation.

> *"If possible, so far as it depnds on you, be at peace with all men."*
>
> Romans 12:18

DAILY REFLECTION

Spend today before God and seek to hear Him in the area of your relationships. Our walk with Him is always reflected in our relationships with others.

_____

_____

_____

_____

Day 5

A New Garment

Today we want to introduce the garment, the lifestyle, which people see when we are being *"strengthened in the inner man by the Spirit of God."* There can be no doubt that Paul is pointing the Ephesians to their lifestyle, their walk in Ephesians 4:17-24, as follows:

> *"This I say therefore, affirm together with the Lord, that you walk no longer just as the Gentiles also walk, in the futility of their mind, being darkened in their understanding, excluded from the life of God, because of the ignorance that is in them, because of the hardness of their heart; and they, having become callous, have given themselves over to sensuality, for the practice of every kind of impurity with greediness. But you did not learn Christ in this way, if indeed you have heard Him and have been taught in Him, just as truth is in Jesus, that, in reference to your former manner of life, you lay aside the old self, which is being corrupted in accordance with the lusts of deceit, and that you be renewed in the spirit of your mind, and put on the new self, which in the likeness of God has been created in righteousness and holiness of the truth."*

Verse 17 talks about us walking no longer just as the Gentiles also walk. Paul then goes on to explain how they walk—in the futility of their minds! In this verse, *mataiotes* is the word translated "futility." In context, it implies the emptiness or the vanity of Gentile minds. The word "mind" comes from *nous*, referring to that part of us that understands or thinks. The word "Gentiles" is translated from *ethnos*, which we get the word "ethnic" from. But in this context, *ethnos* is referring to the pagan, lost world. Now, how do the people who do not know Christ walk? What is their measure of thinking?

When Paul talks of the Gentiles being darkened in their understanding in verse 18, the phrase *"being darkened"* in the Greek is in the perfect passive voice. In New Testament Greek grammar, the perfect tense refers to an action in the past that determines the state of being one is in at the present time. What happened in the past that causes the minds of the pagan world to be darkened?

Read Romans 5:12 and write it below.

_____

_____

_____

The word for "excluded" here is *apallotrioō*. It means to be estranged, alienated, or separated. A lost person is excluded from the life of God. The sin of Adam that was passed on to all humanity caused us all to be estranged and separated from the "life of God." When did we get the "life of God" back?

_____

_____

_____

_____

Paul now shows an attitude that causes the lost world to be held back from receiving the life of God. He mentions the ignorance that is within them. Ignorance comes from the word *agnoia*, meaning a lack of understanding. From this verse, why would there be a lack of understanding?

_____

_____

_____

_____

_____

"Because of the hardness of their hearts!" The word "hardness" refers to something that has become calloused. What does this say to you about those who do not understand and do not have the life of God in them?

_____

_____

_____

_____

Paul continues by saying that they have become callous, *"have given themselves over to sensuality, for the practice of every kind of impurity with greediness."* The phrase *"have become callous"* builds on the former thought. It means that they have grown to be without feeling. *"Have given themselves over to sensuality"* is in the aorist active tense. They of their own choosing have given over themselves. In other words, they have placed themselves alongside with full permission to *"sensuality."* This word for *"sensuality"* is the word *aselgia*. It means a life of wanton living. Anything goes. Pleasure at any cost. The result? *"For the practice of every kind of impurity with greediness."*

Now write out what you have learned about those who have separated themselves from the life of God.

_____

_____

_____

_____

_____

_____

What kind of lifestyle do they live? This was not the way we were instructed to live! Paul says in verse 20 that we did not learn Christ in this way. Look at Ephesians 3:16-17a and Ephesians 4:1-3. How are we to live?

_____

_____

_____

_____

Read Ephesians 4:22. The phrase *"in reference to your former manner of life"* refers to our former lifestyle before Christ. This verse does not contradict Colossians 3:9-11. Read these verses and note that the *"old man"* was put to death when we were saved. Paul is saying to stop living as if the old man hadn't been put to death!

DAILY REFLECTION

When we choose not to be strengthened in the inner man by the Spirit of God, what happens to our relationships to others? You see, by choosing to surrender to Christ, to yield to Him, we put on a new garment. A new lifestyle that others will notice. What does it look like? Well, that's the next lesson. Take a moment to write out what God has spoken to you in our lesson today.

_____

_____

_____

_____

_____

_____

_____

_____

LESSON 6

OUR NEW GARMENT IN CHRIST

Look around at what is going on in our world today, and you see what is flaunted as intelligent and acceptable. Then you compare that with Ephesians 4:17–24; doesn't it burden you for those who do not understand? They cannot understand unless God breaks through their hardened hearts and reveals Himself. But even sadder, is for a believer to live as if he or she thinks the way the world does. Paul is exhorting the Ephesian believers to put on a "new garment." It is put on from the inside out. Christ must strengthen us in the inner man before we are able to walk worthy of that which is ours in Him.

What does this new garment or this new lifestyle look like? That is our lesson this week. We are going to study Ephesians 4:22–32. Actually, this teaching extends through verse 9 of chapter 6, but for the sake of this study we are only going to look at chapter 4. Let's get to it.

DAY 1

DESTINED TO BE LIKE GOD

Read Ephesians 4:22–32 and let's start out by looking at verse 22. Notice that the old self is in a continual state of decline. The phrase "being corrupted" as used here comes from the Greek *phtheirō* meaning to be in a continual state of corruption. An example would be something that has been in the refrigerator for too long and has spoiled. It is getting more and more rotten the longer it sits there.

People who are lost don't realize it, but their lifestyles are getting more and more rotten, and the decay cannot be stopped unless God stops it. But, we have taken that garment off when we were born from above.

Verse 23 says, *"that you have been renewed in the spirit of your mind."* Since we have taken off the "old self," we are now to be renewed in the spirit of our minds. The Greek word translated "renewed" is *ananeoō*. This is the same word used in Romans 12:2. It means to be renovated. Think of something you or someone you know has renovated. What had to be torn out? What had to be added? Now, applying this to the spiritual life, what does this truth say to you?

He goes on to say in verse 24 to, *"put on the new self, which in the likeness of God has been created in righteousness and holiness of the truth."* We are to put on the new self. A new garment is to be put on. A new lifestyle is now ours. Read Ephesians 3:16–17a and note how this new garment is to be put on.

This new lifestyle, new garment, or new self, is destined to be like God! He says, *". . . which in the likeness of God has been created in righteousness and holiness of the truth."* There is no way you and I can act like God unless God Himself produces His life and His likeness in and through us. It begins inward and shows up externally as a lifestyle. This new life is Christ living in and through us. Now read Galatians 2:20 and write this verse below.

DAILY REFLECTION

Now, as our minds are renewed and as the Spirit of God strengthens us in the inner man, we change! Are you changing? What is your lifestyle right now? Take some time to meditate on the passage in Ephesians 4 that we studied today. Pray and ask God to convict you of things in your life that need to be changed by Him. Just as our old self is in a continual state of decay, our new self in Him should be in a continual state of growth and change. Let Him minister His Word to you now.

DAY 2

CHARACTERISTICS OF THE NEW LIFE

Ephesians 4:25 says, *"Therefore, laying aside all falsehood, speak truth, each one of you, with his neighbor, for we are members of one another."* Now, I always say, whenever you see a "therefore" take a look to see what it's there for! (By the way, you just studied it yesterday in case you forgot!) Paul speaks of how the old garment, or old lifestyle, behaved.

Let's begin a list and see its contrast.

First, the Old Self would lie in a minute to protect its image!

Look back at verse 25. There can be no transparency with one another when the old garment is being worn. It is only worn when we choose not to be strengthened in the inner man through our willingness to surrender to Him. We must protect our identity, our reputation. We will lie like a dog when we wear the wrong garment. But, in contrast, when the New Garment is worn, we will speak "truth" with our neighbor because we realize that we are members of one another.

Give an example from your own life when you lied to protect yourself while all the time you knew you were guilty.

_____

_____

_____

_____

Second, the Old Self has the wrong kind of anger.

Verse 26 says, *"Be angry, and yet do not sin; do not let the sun go down on your anger."* Now, is all anger wrong? James 1:20 says that *"the anger of man does not achieve the righteousness of God."* This tells us that there is an anger of man. So then, what are the two types of anger we can have?

_____

_____

How do we tell the difference? Well, if it's the anger of man, then you have the person as your target. But, if it's the anger of God, then you will have the problem as your target. John 3:16 says, "God so loved the world . . . ."

What was the world full of? _____

He hated the sin, but He loved the sinner so much that He sent His Son to come and die for sinners. With God's love being produced in you, you will love the sinner but you will hate and be very angry at the sin. So then, with this in mind, how can you tell when a believer is not wearing the right garment?

_____

_____

_____

Third, the Old Self plays right into the devil's hands.

Verse 27 says, *"and do not give the devil an opportunity."* The Greek word translated "opportunity" is translated "place" in most other instances. This has led many believers to the erroneous view that a believer can have a demon indwell them. They believe that this verse proves that the devil can get into a believer's life and have a "place."

But, as you will notice, the translation here is not "place" but "opportunity." How do you unlock this? Well, it's pretty simple. If you can find other places where the Greek word does not mean "place," then you have an argument where the context should rule. Acts 25:16 and Hebrews 8:7 are two places where this is true.

The context of chapter 4 of Ephesians is "unity of the Body." The Greek word often translated "devil" is the word *diabolos*, with "dia" meaning "through" and "bolos" meaning to cast, to cast through, or to "divide." The devil cannot be in every place at every time. He is not omnipresent. But, we do his bidding when we choose to wear the old garment. We become divisive to the Body, which is Satan's purpose. Are you divisive in the Body of Christ because you refuse to be strengthened in the inner man?

DAILY REFLECTION

Well, what have you learned about the lifestyle that Christ lives through us? It is pretty obvious when we are not wearing the right garment isn't it? Pray and ask God to strengthen you in the inner man and to help you continually to put on the New Garment.

DAY 3

MORE CHARACTERISTICS OF THE NEW LIFE

What have you learned so far about the lifestyle produced when we are living surrendered to Christ, accommodating Him in our hearts?

To review, we first saw that the Old Self is not worried about telling a lie. Second, the Old Self has the wrong kind of anger. And third, the Old Self plays right into the devil's hands.

The fourth characteristic of the old life is that it refuses to give to others.

Verse 28 says, *"Let him who steals steal no longer; but rather let him labor, performing with his own hands what is good, in order that he may have something to share with him who is in need."*

Now, for the sake of our study about the old lifestyle and the contrast the Spirit makes in our lives, let's jump to the main point of the verse. A person who steals is a taker. He takes what is not his and what he has not worked for from someone else. But, he is instructed to work. Why? So that he will have something to give to others.

You see there are two kinds of people. Some who deplete and others who replenish. When we wear the right garment, we will give to others in their need. Selfishness is the mark of one's flesh. Are you a giver or a taker?

Fifthly, the Old Self never edifies others with what is said.

Verse 29 says, *"Let no unwholesome word proceed from your mouth, but only such a word as is good for edification according to the need of the moment, that it may give grace to those who hear."*

There are two words we need to look at in this verse. They tell the whole story. The first word is the word "unwholesome." It is from the Greek *sapros*, and it means rotten and smelly. This presents the image that there is a sense of rottenness or decay when the old garment is worn. Picture an odor that can be detected a mile off.

But, the other word is "edification." It is translated from the Greek *oikodome*. More literally, it means to build a house. Words that are spoken from a life that is being strengthened in the inner man by the Spirit of God are those that build our brothers, they do not break them. What is your conversation about others and to others like?

Now, let's camp here for a while. James 1:26 says, "If anyone thinks himself to be religious, and yet does not bridle his tongue but deceives his own heart, this man's religion is worthless."

The word for "religion" in this verse is *threskos*. It refers to external works. The picture is so clear. There are many people doing many good things, but these works are not generated from the Spirit, because when you listen to these folks, they tear people apart with their tongues.

Journal your thoughts on this.

DAILY REFLECTION

Studying about the Old Garment can be pretty convicting can't it? The Old Self is so ready to take over, but we have to continue to render it dead. Has God convicted you of anything in your own life? There are so many ways that the Old Garment creeps back on us. Sometimes it happens so fast we aren't even aware of it right away. Write out a prayer to God asking Him to keep you sober in the Spirit, always keeping a short account with Him.

_____

_____

_____

_____

_____

_____

_____

_____

_____

DAY 4

DO NOT GRIEVE THE SPIRIT

Wow! What we think is acceptable doesn't always meet God's criteria does it? Well, in today's lesson, it doesn't slow up, but keeps bearing down so that we might understand what it really looks like when we are willing to surrender to Christ and allow His strengthening in the "inner man."

Verse 30 of Ephesians 4 says, *"And do not grieve the Holy Spirit of God, by whom you were sealed for the day of redemption."* When we fail to surrender to Christ with a yielded heart to Him and to His Word, what does this verse say that we are doing?

_____

_____

Look back at verse 27. What else are we doing when this happens?

_____

_____

The word "grieve" means "to cause sorrow." It's Greek equivalent is in the present tense and suggests the thought, "Do not have the habit of grieving the Holy Spirit." How can a believer get into the habit of grieving the Holy Spirit?

_____

_____

_____

_____

One can form a habit by choosing to live life his own way instead of being strengthened in the inner man by the Holy Spirit (see Ephesians 3:16). Write out an example of how you have grieved those whom you love with just such an attitude.

_____

_____

_____

_____

When our attitude is not to surrender to Christ and to His Word, then what are we doing to His Spirit?

_____

_____

The latter part of verse 30 says, *"by whom you were sealed for the day of redemption."* The Holy Spirit is the mark on you. Remember back from our study in Lesson Four? Don't grieve Him!

DAILY REFLECTION

What habits are in your lives that continually grieve the Holy Spirit? What are you going to do about them? Spend some time alone with the Lord to see if you have a habit of grieving His Spirit.

_____

_____

_____

_____

_____

WALKING IN THE NEW GARMENT

Well, what have you learned this week that helps you in your walk with Christ?

_____

_____

_____

_____

_____

These are the characteristics we have seen of the Old Self.

First, the Old Self would lie in a minute to protect its lifestyle (verse 25).

Second, the Old Self always has the wrong kind of anger (verse 26).

Third, the Old Self, when worn, plays right into the devil's hands (verse 27).

Fourth, the Old Self refuses to give to others (verse 28).

Fifth, the Old Self, when worn as a lifestyle, says things about and to others that are rotten (verse 29).

Sixth, the Old Self, that leads us to live our way instead of surrendering to Christ, grieves the Holy Spirit (verse 30).

Remember, we are to be strengthened by the riches of His glory. (Eph. 3:16).

Verse 31 of Ephesians 4 says, _"Let all bitterness and wrath and anger and clamor and slander be put away from you, along with all malice."_

Before we dig into this verse, I want you to notice how Paul gives this list. He does it backwards from the way Peter does in a similar list. Read 1 Peter 2:1 and write it below.

_____

_____

_____

Now, "malice" in both verses is the fabric of the flesh. Where Peter starts with the fabric and lists the progression of how it works in our lives, Paul starts with the end and works it back to the beginning. He starts with bitterness and works back to malice. It's like he wants us to realize how bad it is first and then go back to the source.

It's going to end in bitterness. The Greek word is _pikria,_ which pictures the sickening bitterness of a poison. In the Wayne Barber translation, it is the acid in your stomach you want to spew on your brother, but it will eat you up before you get a chance. It's a terrible state to be in when it comes to relationships. Is there any of that in your life?

_____

_____

_____

Just before you get to that stage, there is wrath. The Greek word here is *thumos*, meaning explosive anger towards someone. Can you think of times when you have witnessed this in your life?

_____

_____

_____

Just before you explode, there is anger, or *orge*. This is anger that is building and building. It hasn't exploded yet, but it is still quietly seething inside you towards your brother. It won't be long until you explode, and bitterness will set in, thus destroying your ability to relate to your brother. You may not have exploded yet, but is this anger seething inside you towards a brother?

Just before the process starts seething inside you, there is "clamor." This word comes from the Greek, *kraugē*, or "loud shouting." All of this is directed towards someone.

Then, just before you start shouting at your brother, you have talked about him behind his back. This is "slander," a strong word to indicate a tearing down of someone's character.

Now we get down to the root of all of the above. "Malice." You see, when you are not being strengthened in the inner man by the Holy Spirit, when you are not willing to yield to Christ and to His Word, when you are doing things your way, no matter how "good" they may look on the outside, the flesh is dominating, and malice has been formed. Is there any malice in your life towards your brother?

Verse 32 says, *"And be kind to one another, tender-hearted, forgiving each other, just as God in Christ also has forgiven you."* Oh what a difference!

The word for "kind" here is *chrestos*. It has the idea of being useful to one another or serving another. *Eusplagchnos* is the word for "tender–hearted." It refers to kindness and tender sensitivity toward others.

Now, look at the last phrase, *"forgiving each other, just as God in Christ also has forgiven you."* Which garment would you rather wear? Which garment are you wearing? How do you put this garment on? From the outside, or does it have to be put on from the inside?

_____

_____

_____

DAILY REFLECTION

We appropriate Christ and all we have in Him when we bow before Him in His Word. Otherwise, the garment we wear on the outside is that which comes from the flesh and nobody is ever blessed by it. Take a moment to review what you have learned this week. Pray and ask God to burn these truths in your heart.

LESSON 7

SURRENDERING TO GOD

It is absolutely amazing to me that so many Christians are trying to enter a room that they already enjoy. They are seeking blessing, anointing, and power, all which are resident in Christ. When I am surrendered to Him and to His Word, then it is no longer I, but Christ. In Him, I can realize all that is necessary for *"life and Godliness"* as Peter so clearly describes in his second epistle. Second Peter 1:3 says, *"seeing that His divine power has granted to us everything pertaining to life and godliness, through the true knowledge of Him who called us by His own glory and excellence."*

Surrender unlocks the door to all that is ours to be
and do what He desires of us.

We have seen that Christ lives in us. We have seen that we have every spiritual blessing in Him. Surrender unlocks the door to all that is ours so that we may be what He desires of us and do what He desires of us. The Christian life is not a matter of "getting more" once we have received Christ; it is a matter of appropriating what we already have in Christ. We are going to study Joshua 1:1-9 in this week's study. Maybe it will become clearer to you.

DAY 1

ENTERING IN

Joshua 1:1-2 says, "Now it came about after the death of Moses the servant of the LORD that the LORD spoke to Joshua the son of Nun, Moses' servant, saying, 'Moses My servant is dead...' " Man, that must have been quite a day for Joshua! Joshua had been a servant to Moses for forty years. Now, he was to take Moses' place and lead the people into the land of Promise.

The instructions God gives Joshua are so important for us to understand. We are not saying that we can substitute ourselves for Joshua or the people of Israel, the context always rules. God is not talking to us, but to the Israelites. However, we must follow the same plan to enter into what is ours as they entered what God had given them.

We have a "life"; they had a "land." But, look very carefully at the way in which they were to enter that land. Today we will begin to look at God's way that has not changed.

Joshua 1:2b-3 says, *"now therefore arise, cross this Jordan, you and all this people, to the land which I am giving them, to the sons of Israel. Every place on which the sole of your foot treads, I have given it to you, just as I spoke to Moses."*

The Hebrew verb stem of the phrase *"I am giving to them"* implies continuous action. Think "I am in the process of giving to them." This is interesting to me. Read the following verses and note the tense when the land is spoken of.

Genesis 15:18 _____

Numbers 20:12 _____

Numbers 20:24 _____

Numbers 27:12 _____

Numbers 27:50-53 _____

Do you notice a different tense in these verses when it refers to the land? Verse 2 in our text says "I am giving it to them," but these verses say "I have given it to them." What is going on? As I studied this, I noticed something that seemed to clear it up. Read Joshua 1:3, and write it below.

_____

_____

_____

The word "sole" is from the word "kaph" meaning the bare part of the foot. It is that tender part of the bare foot. Now, what is this referring to? Exodus 3:5 says, "Then He said, 'Do not come near here; remove your sandals from your feet, for the place on which you are standing is holy ground." Moses is in front of the burning bush on Mt. Horeb, which was a mountain range in Sinai, and on which Mt. Sinai was one of the summits. God told him to take his shoes off. He was standing on holy ground. This ground was set apart, consecrated unto God.

Read Joshua 5:13-15. When Joshua was willing to consider that every step was holy unto God, then that which he stepped upon was already his. Now read Joshua 1:3 and note the last part of this verse. *"Every place on which the sole of your foot treads I have given it to you, just as I spoke to Moses."*

> According to our willingness to bow before Christ
> and surrender to His will for our lives, then and only then,
> are we able to enter what we already have.

Nothing has changed. According to our willingness to bow before Christ and surrender to His will for our lives, then and only then, are we able to enter what we already have. We have seen in Ephesians what we have. How many believers do you know that are living in what they **already** have? Are you?

DAILY REFLECTION

The people to whom God had given the land were forbidden to enter it for forty years because of disobedience to God. Now, the next generation led by Joshua, had another chance. But, they had to learn to consider every step as holy unto Him. Are there areas of your life where you have not realized God's presence and power in, and is it because you have not been willing to bow before Him? Write what God is saying to you.

DAY 2

ENTERING BY OBEDIENCE

Obedience, which is surrendering to God and to His will, has always been His way of our entering into that which He has promised. Some things just do not change.

John 14:21 says, *"He who has My commandments and keeps them, he it is who loves Me; and he who loves Me shall be loved by My Father, and I will love him, and will disclose Myself to him."* The word "disclose" in this verse comes from the Greek *emphanizō*. It means to reveal oneself to someone, or to appear to someone in person.

Christ manifests Himself in and through the lives of those who choose to yield to Him and to His will. In Joshua 1, the Scripture goes on to say in verse 5 that, *"No man will be able to stand before you all the days of your life. Just as I have been with Moses, I will be with you; I will not fail you or forsake you."* It doesn't say, no man will try to stand before you, but *"no man will be able to stand before you."* Man cannot cause you to be dispossessed of what is yours in Him.

If we consider every step to be holy unto Him, no man can take away what is ours in Him. Write how your wrong reaction to another caused you to miss what God says in His Word is yours. (i.e. the fruit of His Spirit working in the lives of those who yield to Him is love, even for those who treat you wrongly.)

DAILY REFLECTION

God is not a respecter of persons. Just as God had been with Moses, Joshua 1:5 tells us that He would now be with Joshua. This must have encouraged Joshua so much. He had watched when God had empowered Moses and given him supreme wisdom. But, this must have also caused him to fear. God was also the One who told Moses he would not enter the Promised Land because of his disobedience. God honors our faith. He honors our surrender to Him and to His will. Are you yielded to Christ and to His will for you? Do you realize what you are missing by not surrendering to Him? Remember, to obey is to surrender and that is the only way we can enter in to what He has for us. Reflect on what God is saying to you.

_____

_____

_____

_____

_____

_____

_____

_____

_____

_____

_____

DAY 3

YIELDING ALL TO HIM

Look up the following verses and note what they tell us about obedience and what they tell us about the choices we have in whom to obey.

Matthew 6:24

_____

John 3:36

_____

_____

Romans 6:13

_____

_____

Romans 6:16

_____

_____

Romans 12:1

_____

_____

We must understand that presenting ourselves before Him through surrender to His will and Word and obeying Him at any cost, is the only way we will ever participate in that which is ours in Him. Nothing has changed! No man can take anything away from us that God says is ours in Christ, but our wrong response to Him and to His Word causes us not to be able to experience what is ours in Him.

DAILY REFLECTION

Take another look at your life. What areas of your life are not yielded to Him?

_____

_____

_____

_____

Are you willing to bow before Christ and lay your stubborn attitude down?

_____

_____

_____

Read Joshua 7:1-12 and write your insights of how the children of Israel handled Ai and the results.

_____

_____

_____

_____

God gave a remedy beginning in verse 12. How is this relevant to us?

_____

_____

_____

Spend some quiet time alone with Him now and listen to what He might be saying to you.

DAY 4

BE STRONG AND COURAGEOUS

Joshua 1:6 says, *"Be strong and courageous, for you shall give this people possession of the land which I swore to their fathers to give them."*

God told Joshua to be strong and courageous. But, then He tells him how this can take place. Have you ever tried in your own power to be strong and courageous? It doesn't work, does it?

_____

_____

_____

_____

Read Joshua 1:7 and write it below.

_____

_____

_____

_____

What does God tell Joshua to do?

_____

_____

The "law" is God's compass for us.

Look up Psalm 1:1-4. How does this relate?

_____

_____

_____

_____

The word "success" in Joshua 1:7 is the word meaning "to act wisely, or to make correct decisions." God strengthens us according to our willingness to obey His Word and, therefore, make wise decisions.

Joshua 1:8 says, *"This book of the law shall not depart from your mouth, but you shall meditate on it day and night, so that you may be careful to do according to all that is written in it; for then you will make your way prosperous, and then you will have success."*

The word "meditate" in this verse carries the idea of pondering something over and over, and has a more literal meaning of a cow continuously chewing and digesting cud! Does just reading God's Word qualify for "meditating?"

_____

_____

_____

Why would we meditate? Joshua 1:8 has the answer: *"So that you may be careful to do according to all that is written in it; for then you will make your way prosperous, and then you will have success."*

Read verse 9 and write it below.

_____

_____

_____

DAILY REFLECTION

How many times must we read Scripture to understand that the only way to make right choices, the only way to be strong and courageous, the only way to enter and enjoy what is ours, is to yield to choose to obey all that God says! Write out your thoughts on how this applies to your life.

_____

_____

_____

_____

_____

_____

_____

_____

DAY 5

THE ENABLING GRACE OF GOD

Well, now it is time to do some review. Let's see how much we remember from the seven lessons that we have studied. We have been looking at the "enabling grace" of God. We have been pointing to that which only God can do. We have shown that God's power only flows through yielded lives. We have tried to show that we already have everything we need in Christ and we do not get anymore, but must learn to appropriate what we have instead.

Fill in the blanks to see how much you remember.

From Romans 6:6, we learned that our bodies are Bodies of _____.

From Romans 6:14, we learned that we are no longer under the performance mentality of the _____ but are now under the enabling power of God's _____ _____.

From Romans 7, we learned the _____ of trying to live under the performance mentality of the law.

From Ephesians 3:16, we learned that our strength comes from _____ _____.

From Ephesians 1:3, we learned that we already have _____ spiritual blessing in Christ.

From Ephesians 1, we learned of all our _____ in Christ.

From Ephesians 3:17, we learned how to appropriate those riches by _____.

From Ephesians 4 we learned that when we are right with Christ then we are right with _____.

From Philippians 1, we learned that Christ must be our _____.

From Philippians 2, we learned that Christ must be our _____.

From Philippians 3, we learned that Christ must be our _____.

From Philippians 4, we learned that Christ must be our _____.

Do you see what the Scripture teaches? Through obedience we can enter that which we already have, and it's all because of His enabling Grace!

DAILY REFLECTION

What a rich study this has been. Continue to review what you have learned so far, and with a surrendered heart, ask God to make it real in your life!

_____

_____

_____

_____

_____

NOTES

LESSON 8

THE WORKS THAT WILL REMAIN

We have almost finished our journey into discovering the Christ life, the enabling message of God's grace and how it is appropriated. I believe it was Watchman Nee that said many years ago that we live in such a "subnormal state" that when we see something that is "normal," we think it is "abnormal." It is my prayer that this study has somehow caused you to realize who and "whose" you are in Christ. I pray that you have realized that He lives in you to do through you what you could never do apart from Him.

In this week's lesson, we will look at why it is so important to realize that the only "works" that will remain when we stand before Him are those that He empowered.

DAY 1

BUILDERS ATTACHED TO CHRIST

The church at Corinth was in a mess!

Read 1 Corinthians 1:10 and answer this question. Why did Paul not want to join the believers in Corinth?

_____

_____

_____

Now read verse 11. What was going on?

_____

_____

_____

What was the source of these quarrels in verse 12?

_____

_____

_____

Some were attached to _____

Some were attached to _____

Some were attached to _____

And yet some others were attached to _____

Now, read 1 Corinthians 11:18. What do you find?

_____

_____

_____

What does 1 Corinthians 12:25 tell us is the case when the Body of Christ is functioning properly?

_____

_____

_____

Is there anyone or anything that you are "attached to" or yielded to other than Christ?

_____

_____

_____

_____

Do you realize that if there is, then you are part of the problem of division in the Body of Christ?

_____

_____

_____

When jealousy and strife are evident among God's people, what does Paul say that they are in God's sight? (Read 1 Corinthians 3:3)

_____

_____

He lives in you to do through you
what you could never do apart from Him

Note in verse 4 how he connects "being fleshly' with being attached to men and not Christ. In your own words, what he is saying here?

_____

_____

Paul knows that he is only a vessel through which God does His work. Read verses 5-7 and write out in your own words what Paul tells us about anyone who is being used as a vessel.

_____

_____

_____

The tense of the phrase in verse 7 "But God who causes the growth" is present tense. If we are yielded or attached to Christ, we are always...

_____

_____

_____

Now, notice how we are "builders" in verse 10. The narrow context is referring to the teachers, or pastors, that followed Paul in Corinth. But, the broader context is that we are all "builders" when we become believers.

With this in mind, look at verse 12 and note what kind of building materials we have to choose from.

_____

_____

_____

What is the foundation, according to verse 11?

_____

_____

DAILY REFLECTION

Are you attached to anything or anyone other than Christ? Are you part of the division of the "Body"? God desires us to be attached to Him in the building up of His Kingdom. Take some time now to reflect on what you have learned and on what God may be saying to your heart today.

_____

DAY 2

TESTED BY FIRE

According to I Corinthians 3:12, Paul says that there are two sets of materials, each with three ingredients in them.

What are the two sets and their ingredients?

_____

_____

_____

To work in the energy of our flesh would constitute what three things?

_____

_____

_____

To work in the energy of the Spirit would constitute what three things?

_____

_____

_____

The results of only one of these two will last. How will these results be tested (verse 13)?

_____

_____

_____

Now, there is integrity to the Christian life. In this world, sometimes we can't see the "motive" behind many people's "works." But when we stand before God, according to 1 Corinthians 4:5, God will one day "disclose the _____ of men's hearts."

What is the day when our "motives" and our "work" will be tested according to verse 13?

_____

_____

Remember that the "day" is not just a single day, but can be a time period. Look at Philippians 1:6. What day does Paul mention?

_____

_____

What day is mentioned in Philippians 1:10?

_____

_____

What day is mentioned in Philippians 2:16?

_____

_____

We are to look forward to that "day." It is not to be feared. It is not to be confused with the "Day of the Lord" which is a terrible day in the future for unbelievers.

To work in the energy of the Spirit
would constitute things that remain.

Since we are to look forward to it, what does this day begin with for the life of a believer? Could it be that 1 Thessalonians 4:13-18 has something to do with it? Read that passage in 1 Thessalonians and note what is to happen on that day.

_____

_____

_____

_____

_____

_____

Believers are to be "caught up together with them in the clouds to meet the Lord in the air." What would many believers call this? The _____ of the church.

On that day, what will be tested by fire according to 1 Corinthians 3:13?

_____

_____

_____

DAILY REFLECTION

Do you realize that your "work" will be tested one day? Are you walking by faith, or are you faking it? Write down your thoughts.

_____

_____

_____

_____

_____

_____

_____

_____

_____

_____

_____

RIGHTEOUS WORKS OF GOD

How many believers are going to have their work tested by fire? Read 1 Corinthians 3:13 and write it below.

_____

_____

What does the "singular" word for "work" say to you?

_____

_____

Each act of serving constitutes a choice that is going into a _____

_____

It is either wood, _____, or _____, or

It is _____, _____, and _____

Romans 1:17 reads "the righteous man shall live by faith."

One is by faith, the other out of the religious works of the flesh. Why would God want to "test" our work? (verse 14)

_____

_____

Note that there are no "unbelievers" even suggested in this passage. Verse 15 shows us that even if there would be the possibility that someone had "no work" left at all after it had been tested, he is still _____ yet so as through fire.

What does this say to those who say that there is only one judgment and all believers and unbelievers will stand together?

_____

_____

_____

The fire cannot destroy what God initiates and enables. It will stand the test. Look at Romans 1:17. How does a person participate in the righteous works of God that cannot be destroyed by fire?

_____

_____

_____

_____

DAILY REFLECTION

Are you realizing that even though it may look good on the outside, unless your works springs forth from faith in God and His Word, then the fire may destroy it one day? How is your walk with Christ? Are you being renewed by His Word and transformed from within by His Spirit? Then the works that flow from that kind of relationship with Him will last. The devil loves religion; it is what man can do. Christianity is not what a man can do for God, but what God can do through a man. Write your thoughts for today.

_____

_____

_____

_____

_____

_____

_____

_____

_____

_____

_____

DAY 4

PROVEN WORTHY

There are three very important words used in verse 13 of 1 Corinthians 3.

"**evident**" — the word "phaneros" which means to cause something to be manifest, to be made so visible that everyone can see it."

"**show it**" — the word "deloō" which means to declare or to inform. It is also used in 1 Corinthians 1:11.

"**reveal**" — is the word "apokaluptō" which means to "uncover or unveil."

There is coming a Day when everything that we have done will be "tested." Note that we are not being "tested." We were judged on the cross. We are in Him. But, it is our _____ _____ that will be tested by fire.

God's intention towards you on this Day when your work is tested
is not to embarrass but to prove you worthy.

The word for "test" is the word "dokimazō." Turn to 1 Peter 1:7 and note the word in that verse. It is translated the same. This word for "test" is always used in a good sense. It is to prove something genuine or worthy. What does this say to you about God's intention towards you on this Day when your work is tested? Is He out to embarrass you or to "get" you?

_____

_____

_____

_____

The word for "fire" is an interesting word in how we see it elsewhere in the New Testament. Read the following verses and note what you learn about the word "fire."

Hebrews 12:29

_____

_____

Revelation 1:14

_____

_____

Revelation 2:18

_____

_____

What mental pictures appear in your mind when you put what you have learned about "fire" and its relationship with Christ and His judgment and with 1 Corinthians 3:13?

_____

_____

_____

_____

DAILY REFLECTION

Isn't it comforting to know that God doesn't want to test our works to condemn us, but to prove us! If we are accommodating Him in our lives and allowing Him to strengthen us in the inner man, He will be the one empowering our works, and those works will be proven worthy one day. This truth gives us all the more reason to be surrendered to Him. Take some time to reflect on what you have learned.

DAY 5

THE MARVELOUS GRACE OF GOD

Well, today is the last day of our study.

You have persevered for eight weeks in studying about the marvelous grace of God. Look at 2 Timothy 2:1 and write it out below.

Where is "grace" found?

When most people think of grace, they always think of the great doctrines of grace that are so awesome; but, in this course, we haven't been focusing on the doctrines of grace, but on the definition of grace. Grace is God's enabling power. It is totally unmerited and undeserved. I want you today in this last day of study, to write all that you can remember that God has shown you about His marvelous grace through this course. Just take your time. After you finish this assignment, take some time to answer the question of what are you going to do about what you have learned.

_____

_____

_____

_____

_____

_____

_____

_____

_____

_____

_____

_____

_____

_____

_____

_____

_____

_____

_____

_____

_____

ADDITIONAL STUDY

Word Study: If you have time, trace the word "fire" through the New Testament and on a separate sheet of paper, write what you discover in the way it characterizes Christ and His judgment.

When you buy a book from **AMG Publishers**, **Living Ink Books**, or **God and Country Press**, you are helping to make disciples of Jesus Christ around the world.

How? AMG Publishers and its imprints are ministries of **AMG** (***Advancing the Ministries of the Gospel***) **International**, a non-denominational evangelical Christian mission organization ministering in over 30 countries around the world. Profits from the sale of AMG Publishers books are poured into the outreaches of AMG International.

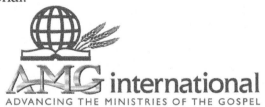

AMG International Mission Statement

AMG exists to advance with compassion the command of Christ to evangelize and make disciples around the world through national workers and in partnership with like-minded Christians.

AMG International Vision Statement

We envision a day when everyone on earth will have at least one opportunity to hear and respond to a clear presentation of the Gospel of Jesus Christ and have the opportunity to grow as a disciple of Christ.

To learn more about AMG International and how you can pray for or financially support this ministry, please visit
www.amginternational.org.

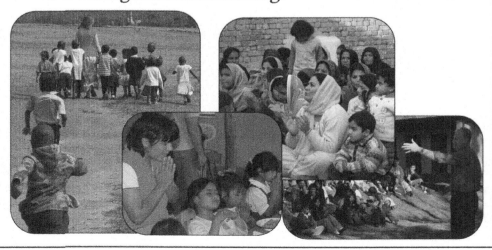

Made in the USA
Coppell, TX
13 December 2019